Health and Human Development Series

CHILDREN AND PAIN

HEALTH AND HUMAN DEVELOPMENT SERIES

JOAV MERRICK, EDITOR

Adolescent Behavior Research: International Perspectives
Joav Merrick and Hatim A. Omar
2007. ISBN: 1-60021-649-8

Complementary Medicine Systems: Comparison and Integration
Karl W. Kratky
2008 ISBN 978-1-60456-475-4

Pain in Children and Youth
Patricia Schofield and Joav Merrick
2008 ISBN 978-1-60456-951-3

Obesity and Adolescence: A Public Health Concern
Hatim A. Omar, Donald E. Greydanus, Dilip R. Patel and Joav Merrick
2009 ISBN 978-1-60456-821-9

Health and Happiness from Meaningful Work: Research in Quality of Working Life
Søren Ventegodt and Joav Merrick
2009 ISBN 978-1-60692-820-2

Behavioral Pediatrics 3rd Edition
Donald E. Greydanus, Dilip R. Patel, Helen D. Pratt and Joseph L. Calles, Jr.
2009. ISBN: 978-1-60692-702-1

Poverty and Children: A Public Health Concern
Alexis Lieberman and Joav Merrick
2009 ISBN 978-1-60741-140-6

Living on the Edge: The Mythical, Spiritual, and Philosophical Roots of Social Marginality
Joseph Goodbread
2009. ISBN 978-1-60741-162-8

Alcohol-Related Cognitive Disorders: Research and Clinical Perspectives
Leo Sher, Isack Kandel and Joav Merrick (Editors)
2009. ISBN 978-1-60741-730-9

Children and Pain
Patricia Schofield and Joav Merrick (Editors)
2009. ISBN 978-1-60876-020-6

Health and Human Development Series

CHILDREN AND PAIN

PATRICIA SCHOFIELD
AND
JOAV MERRICK
EDITORS

Nova Biomedical Books
New York

Library of Congress Cataloging-in-Publication Data

Children and pain / [edited by] Patricia Schofield.
p. ; cm.
Includes index.
ISBN 978-1-60876-020-6 (hardcover)
1. Pain in children--Treatment. 2. Sickle Cell Anemia--Treatment. 3. Pain--Measurement. I. Schofield, Pat (Patricia A.)
[DNLM: 1. Pain--therapy. 2. Adolescent. 3. Anemia, Sickle Cell--drug therapy. 4. Child. 5. Pain Measurement. WL 704 C5355 2009]
RJ365.C45 2009
618.92'0472--dc22

2009027058

Published by Nova Science Publishers, Inc. ✝ New York

Contents

I. Introduction

In: Children and Pain
Editors: P. Schofield and J. Merrick

ISBN 978-1-60876-020-6

Children and pain

Patricia Schofield and Joav Merrick

For many years it was believed that children and in particular babies did not feel pain. But over the last twenty years or so this perspective has changed and we have seen many highly specialised pain clinics being set up around the world, who are dedicated to address the needs of the younger members of the population. Thus acknowledging that children in pain are not simply "smaller adults", but that they have particular experiences and requirements that can only be addressed by experts in the field, who are aware of the developmental factors that may influence their pain experience.

The age of the child, past experience with pain, family and cultural aspects influence the child's response to new, painful situations. The reaction of parents are important and can serve as role models, but also gender differences are important, when it comes to pain in children. Children experience pain often as can be seen from pain diaries with episodes of headaches, abdominal pains, ear pain and limb pains, even several times a week. Chronic persistent pain and disability is less common in children than adults.

The Hospital for Sick Children affiliated with the University of Toronto (www.sickkids.ca/default.asp) has ten ways to ease pain in children:

- Pain should not go untreated, since untreated pain causes stress and can sensitize a child's pain pathways making future bouts of pain worse.
- Assessing the child's pain is the first step to good pain management. Ask how much it hurts (small amount, medium amount or a lot) and what the pain is on a scale from zero to 10, where zero is no pain and 10 is the worst pain you can imagine.
- Remember the three Ps. Depending on the cause, type and severity of pain in your child, you can use a combination of pharmacological therapies (medication) and physical and psychological techniques for pain relief. For example, it is often helpful to combine pain-relieving medication with physical strategies, such as applying heat or ice, and psychological strategies, such as distraction andcontrolled breathing, for pain control.
- Prevention is better than treatment. It is important to give pain medicines regularly to get on top of the pain and to prevent it from becoming unmanageable. There are a

variety of over-the-counter medications that can be effective in treating mild to moderate pain. You should always be cautious when giving medications to children, so ask your pharmacist for help in selecting a medication and how and when to give it to your child.

- The use of cold water and ice can be very helpful in reducing pain. Running cool water over a scrape or minor cut will not only help clean the wound, it will also cool the burning pain. A cool cloth on your child's forehead can help with a headache. Ice is immediately effective in relieving pain caused by bruising, muscle spasms and pulls, sprains and insect stings, as it acts like a mild local anaesthetic. Alternating ice and heat can also be an effective pain relief strategy for swelling, muscle spasms and sore joints.
- Warm baths, warm water bottles and heating pads can also be helpful. Applying heat increases blood flow and can be effective in relieving your child's stiff muscles and joints, bruising and sprains.
- Massage can be helpful with painful muscle spasms and pulls. The sense of touch itself, especially amother touching an infant in pain, is helpful in reducing a child's anxiety and pain.
- Gentle exercise can be useful to help protect muscles from injury and encourage healing in injured areas. A physiotherapist can provide education and instruction on the most appropriate techniques for your child.
- Distraction is a simple and veryeffective way to reduce pain for infants and children. Distraction tends to work best for mild pain and how you distract your child will depend on his age. Babies can be distracted with colourful mobiles and mirrors. Younger children can be distracted with blowing bubbles, reading a favourite book or playing with a musical toy. Older children can choose what they wish to be distracted with, such as a hand-held video game.
- When to seek medical advice. This can be difficult. It is the child who feels the pain of an injury, yet it is up to the caregiver to determine how serious the problem is. The bottom line is that if you are worried about your child's pain, it is reasonable to seek medical attention.

This is sound advice and great for everyday pain, but in this book we will deal with more severe pain in children and pain associated with disease.

Senior lecturer Patricia Schofield, PhD
Centre for Advanced Studies in Nursing, Department of General Practice and Primary Care, University of Aberdeen, United Kingdom. E-mail: p.a.schofield@abdn.ac.uk

Professor Joav Merrick, MD, MMedSci, DMSc
National Institute of Child Health and Human Development, Office of the Medical Director, Ministry of Social Affairs, Jerusalem, Israel and Kentucky Children's Hospital, University of Kentucky, Lexington, United States. E-mail: jmerrick@zahav.net.il

II. Approach to pain

In: Children and Pain
Editors: P. Schofield and J. Merrick
ISBN 978-1-60876-020-6

Chapter 1

Psychological and alternative approaches to pediatric pain

Jennie CI Tsao**, PhD, Qian Lu, MD, PhD and Lonnie K Zeltzer, MD
Pediatric Pain Program, Department of Pediatrics,
David Geffen School of Medicine at UCLA,
Los Angeles, California,
United States of America

Abstract

This chapter highlights recent studies on novel psychological and complementary and alternative medicine (CAM) approaches for acute/procedural and chronic/recurrent pediatric pain. Computerized databases were searched from 1996-2006 to identify controlled trials on CAM therapies and psychological interventions that extended beyond traditional cognitive-behavioral therapy (CBT), defined as clinic-based individual (therapist-child) psychotherapy. Existing data supports the efficacy of novel psychological therapies for both acute and chronic pain reduction. Computer-based and distance (e.g., internet/phone) interventions have emerged as inexpensive new modes of treatment delivery. Well-conducted studies on CAM approaches are limited. Evidence supporting biofeedback for recurrent headaches and hypnosis for acute/procedural pain is the most robust. Compared to the literature on novel psychological interventions, there are relatively few rigorously conducted CAM investigations and thus further well-designed trials are warranted. For novel psychological approaches, additional large-scale studies are needed to replicate initial positive findings.

* Correspondence: Jennie CI Tsao, PhD, Pediatric Pain Program, Department of Pediatrics, David Geffen School of Medicine at UCLA, 10940 Wilshire Blvd., Suite 1450, Los Angeles, CA 90024, United States. Tel: 310-824-7667; Fax: 310-824-0012; E-mail: jtsao@mednet.ucla.edu

Introduction

In the past 20 years, an extensive body of literature has demonstrated that cognitive behavioral therapy (CBT) can benefit pediatric patients with acute or chronic pain. CBT has been designated a "well-established treatment" for procedural pain in children (1) and systematic reviews/meta-analyses support the efficacy of CBT in ameliorating chronic/recurrent pain including headache (2), sickle cell disease (3), and recurrent abdominal pain (4). Researchers have now begun to investigate novel psychological approaches incorporating elements of CBT but going beyond traditional clinic-based CBT in which a therapist treats a child individually. There has also been a burgeoning interest in complementary and alternative medicine (CAM) approaches for pediatric pain (5). CAM has been defined as therapies not generally provided by hospitals and clinics, nor widely taught in medical schools (6).

The purpose of this article is to highlight key findings from recent studies investigating novel psychological and CAM approaches for pediatric pain. Most existing reviews have focused on a single chronic pain condition or only one type of pain (e.g., procedural pain). This article aims to bring together studies on a wide range of pain complaints, including both chronic/recurrent pain and acute/procedural pain in order to provide a broad overview of the field. The intent is to call attention to the advantages and disadvantages of these novel approaches and to identify critical issues in planning future research. PubMed and PsychInfo databases were searched from 1996 to 2006 using the terms, "child," "children," and "pain" to identify relevant studies. Due to the lack of information on randomization among CAM trials, studies with a control group were included even if they did not use randomization or if randomization could not be determined. Effect sizes could not be calculated for the majority of CAM studies and thus were not included. Trials examining novel psychological approaches representing an extension of traditional CBT, defined as clinic-based individual (therapist-child) psychotherapy were included. The following delivery systems are discussed below: brief interventions testing a single component of CBT vs. a complete CBT treatment package; use of parent and nurse coaches (vs. psychotherapists); new technologies (e.g., computers). CAM interventions that have been the subject of at least one controlled trial were also included. Within the two broad categories (i.e., Novel Psychological Approaches; CAM Approaches) studies are grouped according to whether the intervention was used for chronic/recurrent or acute/procedural pain. Within pain categories, studies examining similar types of interventions (e.g., computer-based) are grouped together.

Novel psychological approaches: Acute/procedural pain

Brief memory-based interventions for procedural pain

Traditional CBT involves multiple components delivered over several sessions. In a departure from this time-intensive approach, Chen et al (7) evaluated a brief intervention aimed at reframing negative memories in 50 children (3-18 years) with leukemia during 3 consecutive lumbar punctures (LPs). Relative to controls, children in the intervention group reported reductions in anticipated pain before the second LP, reductions in pain and distress during the third LP, and more positive memories of their previous LP's. More recently, Salmon and colleagues (8) tested a brief intervention employing a cartoon video for procedural pain in 62 children (2-7 years) without chronic medical conditions undergoing a VCUG (voiding cysto-urethrogram, a radiological diagnostic test of the urinary tract and requiring catheterization). Children were randomly assigned to receive complete procedural information (CPI) with cartoon video, limited procedural information (LPI) with cartoon video, or standard care with LPI. Compared to LPI standard care, children in the CPI condition were less distressed during the procedure and appraised the procedure as less painful a week after the procedure. No differences were found between the two LPI conditions. These results suggest that a simple memory-based intervention is efficacious for reducing procedural pain, and that children's memories play an important role in their experience of procedure-related pain and anxiety.

Distraction training: Parents and nurses as "coaches" during immunization

Distraction is defined as any intervention intended to focus the subject's attention away from pain or discomfort; it has been shown to be an effective technique for managing pain related to medical procedures (9). Cohen and colleagues have conducted a series of investigations on distraction interventions for immunization pain provided by parents and nurses. In the first study, they assigned 92 children (4-6 years) to a nurse coach intervention, a nurse coach plus parent coach intervention, or standard care (10). The intervention consisted of children viewing a cartoon movie and being coached to attend to the movie. Compared to the control condition, in the two intervention conditions, children coped more and were less distressed; nurses and parents exhibited more coping-promoting behavior and less distress-promoting behavior. However, the two interventions did not differ on any of the outcome variables. The Cohen group (11) also tested the effectiveness of movie distraction on immunization distress in 136 infants (1-21 months)(12). Parents in the distraction group were briefly trained to redirect the infant's attention to the movie using animated gestures or speech. The distraction group displayed fewer distress behaviors than the standard care group, suggesting that a simple distraction intervention for parents can provide some distress relief to infants during routine injections.

Cohen and colleagues (13) provided 31 children (3-7 years) with brief training in breathing and positive self-statements prior to immunization in the absence of trained nurse or parent coaching, compared to 30 children who did not receive training. Although children understood the training, they did not use the coping strategies during the procedure, suggesting that such training in young children might be insufficient without the inclusion of adult coaches. On the other hand, a study of 69 older children (7-12 years) found that watching a TV cartoon reduced venipuncture pain even more than a mother distraction or control condition. Whereas this study might suggest that parent involvement is not needed if there is a good distractor, the mothers were not trained in how to distract their child. One tentative conclusion is that training of parents to improve distraction skills in children might be necessary for maximal benefits (14).

Virtual reality as a distraction tool for acute and procedural pain

New developments in media technology, such as virtual reality (VR), computers, and the internet, create unprecedented opportunities to deliver pain management programs for children in alternative, efficient ways. Growing up with these new technologies, children and adolescents may be particularly receptive to interventions using these techniques. VR is an exciting new approach that has recently been used as a distraction method in managing acute and procedural pain. In a preliminary study with seven children (5-6 years) with acute burn injuries (15), VR combined with routine pharmacological analgesia led to lower pain reports than analgesia alone during burn dressing changes. Similarly, in a pilot study of 20 children (8-12 years) (16), VR reduced pain relative to a control condition during pediatric intravenous (IV) placement. VR pain distraction was positively endorsed by children, parents and nurses in both studies. VR as a distraction method appears to be promising and attractive for children, and further studies with larger samples are warranted.

Novel psychological approaches: Chronic/recurrent pain

Computer and internet based interventions

Newer technologies for treatment delivery have also been tested for chronic/recurrent pain. Connelly et al (17) examined the effects of a CD-ROM program in 37 children (7-12 years) with recurrent headache. Treatment consisted of a CD-ROM program (including education, relaxation, thought-changing, and pain behavior modification) self-administered on home computers. Children in the CD-ROM group evidenced significant improvements in headache activity compared to controls by 3-month follow-up. Although encouraging, these finding require replication in a larger sample.

Distance methods have considerable potential for making effective treatments more accessible with lower associated costs. Hicks (18) examined distance treatment delivered via internet and telephone in 47 children (9–16 years) with recurrent headache or abdominal pain. The intervention employed a Web-based manual with CBT techniques (e.g., relaxation; cognitive strategies) with weekly therapist contact by telephone or e-mail. The control group was a standard medical care waitlist group who were reminded to see their physician as needed. At the 1- and 3-month follow-ups respectively, 70% and 72% of the treatment group achieved clinically significant improvement (50% reduction in pain), whereas only 19 and 14% of the control group achieved the criterion. With an average treatment time per participant of approximately 3 hours, the distance treatment was estimated to be 5.5 times more cost-effective in the consumption of therapist time than office-based individual therapy.

Nevertheless, 35% of patients who expressed initial interest in the study did not complete baseline measures suggesting that attrition may be high for such distance interventions.

CAM approaches for pediatric pain: Acute/procedureal pain

Music for procedural pain

In contrast to these new technologies, music has been used since antiquity to enhance well-being (19). Two types of music-based interventions for procedural pain have been studied: 1) music therapy involving the live performance of trained therapists; 2) recorded music. The extent to which these modalities can be clearly differentiated is unclear. Music is thought to function as a form of distraction that may indirectly influence pain (20). Nevertheless, few studies have tested whether music offers any specific analgesic benefits by including placebo conditions to control for non-specific effects due to other types of distraction.

Mixed results on the benefits for music for procedural pain have been reported. Megel et al. (21) in 99 children (3 – 6 years) found that those who listened to lullabies during immunization displayed less distress relative to no intervention controls, although the groups did not differ in physiological responses or reported pain. However, this study suffered from serious methodological limitations including lack of information regarding randomization and how the distress ratings were conducted. Malone (22) tested the effects of live music therapy for pain related to intravenous starts, venipunctures, injections and heel sticks in 20 children (0-7 years) and 20 no intervention controls, matched for age and type of needle insertion. The music group displayed less behavioral distress than controls during pre- and post-needle stages, although there were no group differences in distress during needle insertion. This study suffered from the same limitations as the Megel study regarding randomization and distress ratings. Null findings have also been reported. A very recent study found no significant differences in injection pain among 64 children (4 to 6.5 years) who listened to either music or a story while pointing to pictures, compared to no intervention controls (23). In accord, a recent Cochrane review (24) including 51 studies (eight pediatric) of music for pain relief concluded that although music reduced pain, the magnitude of the reductions was small and thus the relevance of music for clinical practice remains unclear.

Hypnosis

Hypnosis involves imaginative experiences in which the subject is guided to respond to suggestions for changes in subjective experience and alterations in perception and emotion. It is viewed as particularly appropriate for children due to their increased susceptibility to hypnosis relative to adults (25); this enhanced susceptibility has been attributed to children's willingness to become absorbed in fantasy (26).

Hypnosis for procedural pain in pediatric oncology

Two recent comprehensive reviews have summarized the literature on hypnosis for procedural pain in pediatric cancer (27,28). Despite extensive overlap in the studies included in these reviews, their conclusions diverged. Wild and Espie assigned a grade of "D" to the quality of existing evidence indicating inconsistent results and generally poor methodological quality. The Richardson review was more positive, emphasizing that statistically significant reductions in pain were found despite a number of methodological limitations. These more optimistic conclusions were based in part on the results of Liossi and Hatira (29) who tested a manualized hypnosis intervention for procedural pain in 80 pediatric cancer patients (6-16 years) who received hypnosis, attention control, or standard medical care. Hypnosis resulted in less pain and anxiety relative to both control conditions. This study was methodologically superior to prior studies in that a treatment manual was used and adherence checks for treatment fidelity were conducted by an independent observer. However, there was only one study therapist and thus, additional replication studies are required to determine the generalizability of these findings.

Extending these results Liossi and colleagues (30) randomly assigned 45 pediatric cancer patients (6-16 years) undergoing LPs to receive either eutectic mixture of local anesthetics (EMLA) alone, EMLA plus hypnosis or EMLA plus attention. The hypnosis group demonstrated less distress and reported less anticipatory anxiety and less procedure-related pain and anxiety relative to the other groups. This study possessed several methodological strengths including the use of a treatment manual and good treatment fidelity, as well as high inter-reliability for behavioral observations of distress and data indicating raters were unaware of group assignment. Nevertheless, the use of only one study therapist (the principal investigator) points to the need for further replication in an independent research group.

Hypnosis for procedural pain related to VCUG

Butler et al (31) randomized 44 children (aged 4 -15 years) without chronic medical conditions undergoing VCUG to receive either hypnosis or routine care. Compared to routine care, hypnosis resulted in lower parent ratings of child distress, less child distress as rated by an experimenter, less difficulty in performing the procedure as reported by medical staff, and shorter procedure time. One major limitation of this study is that the medical staff, experimenters and parents were all aware of group assignment.

Hypnosis for pediatric burn-dressing changes

A randomized controlled trial (RCT) on pediatric burn victims (32) examined 23 children (3 - 12 years) who received "familiar imagery" (i.e., imagery related to familiar experiences) or attention control during 3 dressing changes. Hypnosis did not result in decreased distress in the treated group relative to baseline, nor were there any differences between the treated and control groups. Based on these findings, it is unclear whether hypnosis holds promise as an intervention for pain related to pediatric burn-dressing procedures.

Hypnosis for post-operative pain

Lambert (33) found that children (7 to 19 years) who received hypnosis reported significantly lower pain ratings and shorter hospital stays than those given standard care, although the groups did not differ in the amount of pain medication received. In a well-conducted study, Huth et al. (34) randomly assigned 73 children (7 -12 years) to imagery delivered via video- and audio-tapes or attention-control. Post-surgery, the imagery group reported less pain and anxiety than controls. However, this study did not include a placebo group since the authors maintained that children may have distracted themselves in some other way (e.g., watching TV). This consideration highlights an inherent difficulty in devising a suitable placebo condition beyond mere attention to control for non-specific effects in trials of hypnosis.

CAM approaches for pediatric pain: Chronic/recurrent pain

Acupuncture for pediatric migraine

Acupuncture involves the use of needles, heat, pressure or other stimulation at points along the meridian to enhance flow of energy or Qi. Despite the conventional view that children are afraid of needles, uncontrolled studies have demonstrated the feasibility and acceptability of acupuncture for children with chronic pain problems (35). The sole RCT on acupuncture for recurrent pediatric pain (36) compared 22 patients (7-15 years) with migraine headaches who received either true acupuncture, or placebo acupuncture (superficial needling). The true acupuncture group evidenced clear reductions in migraine frequency and severity compared to no improvements in the placebo group. Although the study was rigorously conducted, the sample sizes were relatively small and patients receiving medication were excluded even though many migraine patients are on regular, prophylactic and/or as needed medications, suggesting that the findings may be of limited generalizability. Also, there was no follow-up data so it is unclear whether improvements persisted across time.

Biofeedback for recurrent pediatric headaches

The most frequently studied forms of biofeedback (BFB) are thermal biofeedback (TBF; volitional handwarming) which involves monitoring visual and/or auditory feedback from a thermistor placed on the fingers and electromyographic biofeedback (EMG-BFB) which involves monitoring visual and/or auditory feedback from electric impulses generated from the frontalis muscle. BFB for recurrent headaches has been the subject of numerous reviews [e.g.,(37, 38)] and meta-analyses [e.g., (2, 39)]. The general conclusion of these investigations is that existing research supports the efficacy of BFB for recurrent pediatric headache despite methodological weaknesses such as wide age range of patients, differing or unspecified diagnoses, variation in headache severity and inconsistencies regarding medication usage (39).

Three studies on BFB for recurrent headache have been published in time period covered by this review. Scharff et al (40) compared TBF to a placebo (handcooling) and wait list in 36 children (mean age = 12.8 years) with pediatric migraine. A greater proportion of the TBF group (53.8%) exhibited at least a 50% reduction in symptoms compared to the placebo group (10%) at post-treatment, and 3-, and 6-month follow-ups; there were no changes in the wait list group. This study demonstrated that BFB evidenced analgesic effects beyond that of a credible placebo control. The second study found that 10 children with pediatric migraines (mean age 10.5 years) trained to self-regulate slow cortical potential (SCPs) reported reduced migraine frequency and migraine index (number monthly attacks X severity X duration) compared to 10 no intervention controls (mean age 11.6 years)(41); trained children were significantly more likely to report a >50% reduction in migraine days than control children. Although this study provides preliminary support for self-regulation of SCPs in pediatric migraine, additional work with larger samples is required. The third study (42) compared EMG-BFB to relaxation in 35 children (11 to 15 years) with tension headaches. Although the groups did not differ at 1-month post-treatment, by 6- and 12-month follow-ups, the EMG-BFB group achieved significantly greater symptom reduction compared to controls. Based on this study, it appears that TBF holds promise as an intervention in childhood tension headaches although further carefully controlled studies are needed.

Massage therapy for juvenile rheumatoid arthritis

Massage therapy refers to the manipulation of soft-tissue by trained therapists for therapeutic purposes. In the only RCT examining massage for children with chronic pain (43), 20 children with juvenile rheumatoid arthritis (JRA) (5-14 years) received either a daily 15 minute massage administered by their parents or a daily 15 minute relaxation session with their parents. After 30 days, the massage group experienced less pain according to children, parents and physicians compared to controls. Although this study used standardized massage protocols and assessments by an independent physician, the sample sizes were small and it is unclear how well parents adhered to the massage protocol. Future studies may include control conditions such as sham massage (light touch) to permit investigation of specific effects obtaining to massage while controlling for non-specific effects due to physical contact.

Discussion

Notable advances in the delivery of psychological and CAM treatments for pediatric pain beyond the traditional CBT model have been reported. Regarding novel psychological approaches, brief memory-based interventions represent a less time-intensive yet effective approach for acute procedural pain (7,8). Work by Cohen and colleagues (10,12) supports the use of parents and medical practitioners as cost-effective agents in the management of injection pain. The use of new technologies as treatment delivery systems has also gained support. For acute pain, preliminary work supports the utility of VR as a distraction tool during dressing changes for acute burn injuries (15) and procedural pain related to IV placement (16). For patients with chronic/recurrent pain, computer- and telephone-based interventions with minimal therapist contact have generated therapeutic benefits for children with recurrent headaches (17) and/or abdominal pain (18). These inexpensive approaches may be especially suited for children in rural communities, ethnic minorities, and those of limited economic means. Interventions employing the internet, CD-ROM and portable electronic devices (PDA) create cost-effective opportunities for pain management and potentially allow for outreach to geographically remote locations.

Several potential problems however, exist in conducting distance treatment studies. As discussed above, attrition rates in distance treatment might be higher than those observed in traditional settings. Establishing a good therapist-patient relationship in distance treatment might be more difficult compared to traditional settings. Hicks et al (18) recommended an initial face-to-face office visit to establish rapport and to ultimately combine both traditional and unconventional approaches to maximize effective service delivery resources, especially for distance treatments. Distance treatment may particularly benefit those who have chronic conditions that require multiple treatment sessions and who have difficulty accessing traditional treatment locations. Another caveat to these initial findings is that sample sizes have been relatively small. Future large-scale studies are needed to establish the generalizability of these results for newer technologies.

In general, there have been far fewer rigorously conducted CAM trials for pain compared to the large number of high quality studies examining psychological approaches. For modalities such as acupuncture and massage therapy, which have been the subject of only one controlled trial each, there is insufficient data to draw definitive conclusions regarding efficacy. Recent research on the effects of music for procedural pain has been mixed with some studies reporting positive results (21,22) but at least one recent investigation reporting null findings (23). In contrast, there is good evidence from high quality trials supporting the utility of hypnosis for procedural pain in pediatric oncology (29,30). Hypnosis has also demonstrated therapeutic effects on procedural pain related to VCUG (31) and post-operative pain (33,34), but no such benefits on pain related to burn dressing changes (32). There is also considerable support for the application of BFB for recurrent headaches (39), although fewer studies have focused on tension headaches compared to pediatric migraine. Due to a lack of controlled studies, several CAM interventions, including movement therapies (e.g., yoga), meditation, energy healing, were not discussed in this article. Additional work may be directed at the rigorous testing of these potentially useful CAM modalities for the management of pediatric pain.

Acknowledgments

This chapter was supported in part by R01DE012754, awarded by the National Institute of Dental and Craniofacial Research, and UCLA General Clinical Research Center Grant MO1-RR-00865 (PI: Lonnie K. Zeltzer), and by R01MH063779, awarded by the National Institute of Mental Health (PI: Margaret C. Jacob). Dr. Lu is supported by UCLA Jonsson Comprehensive Cancer Center Postdoctoral Fellowship.

References

[1] Powers SW. Empirically supported treatments in pediatric psychology: procedure- related pain. J Pediatr Psychol 1999:24(2): 131-45.
[2] Eccleston C et al. Systematic review of randomised controlled trials of psychological therapy for chronic pain in children and adolescents, with a subset meta-analysis of pain relief. Pain 2002; 99(1-2):157.
[3] Chen E, Cole SW, Kato PM. A review of empirically supported psychosocial interventions for pain and adherence outcomes in sickle cell disease. J Pediatr Psychol 2004;29(3):197-209.
[4] Janicke DM, Finney JW. Empirically supported treatments in pediatric psychology: recurrent abdominal pain. J Pediatr Psychol 1999;24(2):115-27.
[5] Tsao JCI, Zeltzer LK. Complementary and alternative medicine approaches for pediatric pain: A review of the state-of-the-science. Evid Based Complement Alternat Med 2005;2:149-59.
[6] Eisenberg DM et al. Unconventional medicine in the United States: prevalence, costs, and patterns of use. New Engl J Med 1993;328: 246-52.
[7] Chen E et al. Alteration of memory in the reduction of children's distress during repeated aversive medical procedures. J Consult Clin Psychol 1999;67:481-90.
[8] Salmon K, McGuigan F, Pereira JK. Brief report: Optimizing children's memory and management of an invasive medical procedure: The influence of procedural narration and distraction. J Pediatr Psychol 2006;31(5):522-7.
[9] Kleiber C, Harper D. Effects of distraction on children's pain and distress during medical procedures: A meta-analysis. Nurs Res 1999;48:44-9.
[10] Cohen LL, Blount RL, Panopoulos G. Nurse coaching and cartoon distraction: An effective and practical intervention to reduce child, parent, and nurse distress during immunizations. J Pediatr Psychol 1997;22(3):355-70.
[11] Cohen LL et al. Randomized clinical trial of distraction for infant immunization pain. Pain 2006;125(1-2):165.
[12] Cohen, LL et al. Randomized clinical trial of distraction for infant immunization pain. Pain 2006;125:165-71.
[13] Cohen LL et al. A child-focused intervention for coping with procedural pain: Are parent and nurse coaches necessary? J Pediatr Psychol 2002;27(8):749-57.
[14] Bellieni CV et al. Analgesic effect of watching TV during venipuncture. Arch Dis Child 2006;91(12):1015-7.
[15] Das D et al. The efficacy of playing a virtual reality game in modulating pain for children with acute burn injuries: A randomized controlled trial [ISRCTN87413556]. BMC Pediatrics 2005;5(1):1.
[16] Gold JI et al. Effectiveness of virtual reality for pediatric pain distraction during IV placement. Cyber Psychol Behav 2006;9(2): 207-12.
[17] Connelly M et al. Headstrong: A pilot study of a CD-ROM intervention for recurrent pediatric headache. J Pediatr Psychol 2006;31(7):737-47.
[18] Hicks CL, von Baeyer CL, McGrath PJ. Online psychological treatment for pediatric recurrent pain: A randomized evaluation. J Pediatr Psychol 2006;31(7):724-36.
[19] Kemper KJ, Danhauer SC. Music as therapy. South Med J 2005;98(3):282-8.
[20] Farthing GW, Venturino M, Brown SW. Suggestion and distraction in the control of pain: test of two hypotheses. J Abn Psychol 1984; 93(3):266-76.
[21] Megel ME, Houser CW, Gleaves LS. Children's responses to immunizations: Lullabies as a distraction. Issues in Comprehensive Pediatr Nurs 1999;21:129-45.
[22] Malone AB. The effects of live music on the distress of pediatric patients receiving intravenous starts, venipunctures, injections, and heel sticks. J Music Ther 1996;33:19-33.
[23] Noguchi LK. The effect of music versus nonmusic on behavioral signs of distress and self-report of pain in pediatric injection patients. J Music Ther 2006;43:16-38.

[24] Cepeda MS et al. Music for pain relief. Cochrane Database Syst Rev 2006(2):CD004843.
[25] Milling LS, Costantino CA. Clinical hypnosis with children: first steps toward empirical support. Int J Clin Exp Hypn 2000;48(2): 113-37.
[26] Olson M, Kohen DJ. Hypnosis and hypnotherapy with children, Third ed. New York: Guilford, 1996.
[27] Richardson J et al. Hypnosis for procedure-related pain and distress in pediatric cancer patients: A systematic review of effectiveness and methodology related to hypnosis interventions. J Pain Sympt Manage 2006;31(1):70.
[28] Wild MR, Espie CA. The efficacy of hypnosis in the reduction of procedural pain and distress in pediatric oncology: a systematic review. J Dev Behav Pediatrics 2004;25(3):207-13.
[29] Liossi C, Hatira P. Clinical hypnosis in the alleviation of procedure-related pain in pediatric oncology patients. Int J Clin Exp Hypn 2003;51(1):4-28.
[30] Liossi C, White P, Hatira P. Randomized clinical trial of local anesthetic versus a combination of local anesthetic with self-hypnosis in the management of pediatric procedure-related pain. Health Psychol 2006;25(3):307-15.
[31] Butler LD et al. Hypnosis reduces distress and duration of an invasive medical procedure for children. Pediatrics 2005;115(1):e77-85.
[32] Foertsch CE et al. Treatment-resistant pain and distress during pediatric burn-dressing changes. J Burn Care Rehabil 1998;19(3):219-24.
[33] Lambert SA. The effects of hypnosis/guided imagery on the postoperative course of children. J Dev Behav Pediatrics 1996; 17(5):307-10.
[34] Huth MM, Broome ME, Good M. Imagery reduces children's post-operative pain. Pain 2004;110(1-2):439-48.
[35] Zeltzer LK et al. A phase I study on the feasibility of an acupuncture/hypnotherapy intervention for chronic pediatric pain. J Pain SymptManage 2002;24:437-46.
[36] Pintov S et al. Acupuncture and the opioid system: implications in management of migraine. Pediatr Neurol 1997;17(2):129-33.
[37] Hermann C, Blanchard EB. Biofeedback in the treatment of headache and other childhood pain. Appl Psychophysiol Biofeedback 2002;27(2):143-62.
[38] Holden EW, Deichmann MM, Levy JD. Empirically supported treatments in pediatric psychology: recurrent pediatric headache. J Pediatr Psychol 1999;24(2):91-109.
[39] Trautmann E, Lackschewitz H, Kroner-Herwig B. Psychological treatment of recurrent headache in children and adolescents--a meta-analysis. Cephalalgia 2006;26(12):1411-26.
[40] Scharff L, Marcus DA, Masek BJ. A controlled study of minimal-contact thermal biofeedback treatment in children with migraine. J Pediatr Psychol 2002;27(2):109-19.
[41] Siniatchkin M et al. Self-regulation of slow cortical potentials in children with migraine: an exploratory study. Appl Psychophysiol Biofeedback 2000;25(1):13-32.
[42] Bussone G et al. Biofeedback-assisted relaxation training for young adolescents with tension-type headache: a controlled study. Cephalalgia 1998;18(7):463-7.
[43] Field TM et al. Juvenile rheumatoid arthritis: benefits from massage therapy. J Pediatr Psychol 1997;22(5):607-17.

In: Children and Pain
Editors: P. Schofield and J. Merrick
ISBN 978-1-60876-020-6

Chapter 2

Treating chronic pain in children from a holistic point of view

***Søren Ventegodt, MD, MMedSci, EU-MSc*[*1,2,3,4,5] and**
***Joav Merrick, MD, MMedSci, DMSc*[6,7,8]**
[1]Quality of Life Research Center, Classensgade 11C, 1 sal,
DK-2100 Copenhagen O, Denmark
[2]Research Clinic for Holistic Medicine
[3]Nordic School of Holistic Medicine, Copenhagen, Denmark
[4]Scandinavian Foundation for Holistic Medicine, Sandvika, Norway
[5]Interuniversity College, Graz, Austria
[6]National Institute of Child Health and Human Development
[7]Office of the Medical Director, Division for Mental Retardation,
Ministry of Social Affairs, Jerusalem, Israel
[8]Kentucky Children's Hospital, University of Kentucky, Lexington, United States

Abstract

Holistic medicine consider the human being as body, mind and spirit. These three parts contain a core talent: sexuality, consciousness and love. To function healthy the child needs to develop the related functions: personal character and gender, verbal and intuitive intelligence, social and emotional capabilities. A child with arrested psychosexual development can deny its gender, have compromised development of language and social intelligence. When meeting the parents in the clinic the reasons for the child's situation normally becomes obvious, since the child is mirroring its parents and the child often functions as the "family's thermometer". Some times chronic pains and also more severe health problems arising from a dysfunctional family patterns can be helped by addressing the problems courageously and openly. When the problems have

[*] Correspondence: Søren Ventegodt, MD, MMedSci, MSc, Director, Quality of Life Research Center, Classensgade 11C, 1 sal, DK-2100 Copenhagen O, Denmark. Tel: +45-33-141113; Fax: +45-33-141123; E-mail: ventegodt@livskvalitet.org

been seen and expressed, the power of them are often reduced significantly, and a new development and healing can start.

Introduction

During the last decades research in holistic medicine and psychodynamic therapy has intensified (1-3). The reason seems to be an understanding that health and diseases is very much a product of psychosocial, quality of life and life-style factors. The approach in pediatrics has always been much more holistic than adult medicine. In pediatrics much of the focus is on thriving and development and the pediatrician use the tools from the traditional holistic medicine - i.e. the holistic medicine going back to Hippocrates and the Greek physicians (4), which in our point of view has been traditionally preserved in this specialty.

Most unfortunately the last decades of development has taken pediatrics much closer to biomedicine and the focus on the whole person and the family diminished, leaving many children with unsolvable problems from unattended psychosocial reasons (5-7).

The triad of poor physical health, especially chronic pain, lack of motivation and other emotional disturbances, and arrested psychosexual development strongly indicates that the problem is of general and existential, "holistic" nature (8). Often an interview with the family will reveal a severely dysfunctional or broken family, and the emotional healing of the wound from lack of sufficient parenting must be the physician or therapists primary focus.

If the child has recurrent physical pain then this is often the best place to start as everybody can agree that this is not right. Most often the parents will deny neglect or abuse of the child, whether this is psychic and emotional, physical or sexual. The parents and other central family member interaction with the child must be observed closely, and small and symbolic expressions of neglect and abuse must be addressed in the therapy, and the meaning and significance of concrete examples must be discussed in the family.

Holistic medicine is consciousness-based medicine (9), and the primary intention with the intervention is to make everybody present aware of what is going on and aware of the reasons why things are happening the way they are, and alternatives sought that could make things work better when being at home.

As a therapist it is often possible to give a good example of contact, communicational and emotional support for the parents and siblings etc. to learn from. Surprisingly often just this can give a complete change in the child's situation, and one single session where the parents got a better idea of parenting and some sound principles that can significantly change the health status of a child.

Body-mind-spirit

Holistic medicine sees man as consisting of body, mind and spirit. These three parts contain a core talent: sexuality, consciousness, and love. To function healthy the child needs to develop the related functions: personal character and gender, verbal and intuitive intelligence, and social and emotional capabilities.

A child with arrested psychosexual development will often deny its sex or not present itself as a "sweet and loving boy or girl"; the development of language will be compromised and social intelligence will typically be poor (8).

When meeting the parents the reasons for the child's situation normally becomes obvious. The child is mirroring its parents, and the child functions as the "family's thermometer", meaning that if the child is ill, the whole family often also is.

Interestingly most even severe health problems arising from even severely dysfunctional families can be helped by addressing the problems courageously and openly (9-11). As soon as the problems have been seen and expressed, the power of the problems are reduced, and a new development and healing starts.

In a family practice things are often neither good nor bad, but many things can be improved and bettered. During the years, when every visit to the doctor leads to a little improvement, some new important insights, and a few new exercises for use at home to improve the family relations, the whole family will grow and improve. The holistic physician can see himself as a gardener taking away some weed every time he passes the roses. As time goes by the roses will start to blossom again.

Chronic stomach pain or for example chronic knee pain can be supported with gentle massage to intensify the contact between patient and physician, and gentle exercises for home use can be given, as a way for the parents or siblings to give physical care and attention to the child (12-14). Everything that gets the sensation of allowing love to be expressed will help the child, for love is what every child in the end most importantly needs to be cured through the process of salutogenesis (15,16).

Conclusions

Children are more susceptible to somatisation than adults, and therefore psychosocial intervention is often more efficient with children. If the physician or holistic therapist is able to pinpoint the dysfunctional family patterns in such a way that the parents understands what is wrong and make corrections to improve the situation, the child will often benefit significantly.

It is most important for the parents to understand fully that what children needs for growth, development and thriving is love, care, acceptance, awareness and respect for their individuality and personal character. The physician has a unique platform to demonstrate these parenting qualities, and when this is done poor thriving, arrested development and chronic pain and other health problems can often be alleviated.

Most often when it comes to sick kids, the key for healing and improvement is not blood tests, weighing and measuring and similar clinical procedures, but just the physician being with the child and his family, helping them to understand their life and the dynamics of the family situation.

The physician should not neglect his duties of physical examination, but always remember that for a child love and care means more that healthy food and exercise for health and quality of life.

References

[1] Leichsenring F, Rabung S, Leibing E. The efficacy of short-term psychodynamic psychotherapy in specific psychiatric disorders: a meta-analysis. Arch Gen Psychiatry 2004;61(12):1208-16.

[2] Leichsenring F. Are psychodynamic and psychoanalytic therapies effective? A review of empirical data. Int J Psychoanal 2005;86(Pt 3):841-68.

[3] Leichsenring F, Leibing E. Psychodynamic psychotherapy: a systematic review of techniques, indications and empirical evidence. Psychol Psychother 2007;80(Pt 2):217-28

[4] Jones WHS. Hippocrates. Vol. I–IV. London: William Heinemann, 1923-1931.

[5] Ventegodt S. Every contact with the patient should be therapeutic. J Pediatr Adolesc Gynecol 2007;20(6):323-4.

[6] Ventegodt S, Morad M, Merrick J. Clinical holistic medicine: developing from asthma, allergy, and eczema. ScientificWorldJournal 2004;4:936-42.

[7] Ventegodt S, Morad M, Press J, Merrick J, Shek DT. Clinical holistic medicine: holistic adolescent medicine. ScientificWorldJournal 2004;4:551-61.

[8] Ventegodt S, Merrick J. The life mission theory IV. Theory on child development. ScientificWorldJournal 2003;3:1294-1301.

[9] Ventegodt S, Merrick J. Clinical holistic medicine: applied consciousness-based medicine. ScientificWorldJournal 2004;4:96-99.

[10] Ventegodt S, Morad M, Hyam E, Merrick J. Clinical holistic medicine: when biomedicine is inadequate. ScientificWorldJournal 2004;4:333-46.

[11] Jung CG. Man and his symbols. New York: Anchor Press, 1964.

[12] Ventegodt S, Merrick J. Clinical holistic medicine: chronic pain in internal organs. ScientificWorldJournal 2005;5:205-10.

[13] Ventegodt S, Merrick J. Clinical holistic medicine: chronic pain in the locomotor system. ScientificWorldJournal 2005;5:165-72.

[14] Ventegodt S, Morad M, Merrick J. Clinical holistic medicine: classic art of healing or the therapeutic touch. ScientificWorldJournal 2004;4:134-47.

[15] Antonovsky A. Health, stress and coping. London: Jossey-Bass, 1985.

[16] Antonovsky A. Unravelling the mystery of health. How people manage stress and stay well. San Franscisco: Jossey-Bass, 1987.

III. Acute pain

In: Children and Pain
Editors: P. Schofield and J. Merrick
ISBN 978-1-60876-020-6

Chapter 3

Acute musculoskeletal sports injury

Amit M Deokar**, MD, MPH, Shawn J Smith, MD and Hatim A Omar, MD, FAAP
Department of Pediatrics, Division of Adolescent Medicine,
University of Kentucky, Lexington, Kentucky, United States

Abstract

The objective of this chapter is to summarize the current standards of pain management in minor sports related musculoskeletal injuries. This article also addresses the topical form of non-steroidal anti-inflammatory drug as an effective pain management option in an out-patient setting. Design: Quantitive systematic review of randomized controlled trials. Methods: The data was obtained through literature review of articles published in the last 10 years. In addition, FDA information on non-steroidal anti-inflammatory medications was also reviewed. The patient population studied in the articles included children and adults. Conclusion: Current standards of managing pain resulting from sports injuries involve a number of analgesic drugs including non-steroidal anti-inflammatory drugs. The topical form of this class of drugs is an effective method for pain management of minor musculoskeletal sports-related injuries.

Introduction

When compared to the 1970's, there has been increased participation in sports activities. Despite an increased awareness of safety measures, the participants are still at an increased risk from sports-related injuries (1). Various agencies are involved in the surveillance and epidemiologic data on sports-related injuries. National Health Interview Survey is one such agency that collects data for the National Center for Health Statistics (NCHS) (2).

Musculoskeletal injuries are one of the primary reasons that patients seek medical attention in the out-patient family practice setting (3). Throughout the United States, a large portion of emergency department (ED) visits is following acute sports-related injuries (4). Approximately 3.7 million sports-related injuries occur in people of all ages and each year about 2.5 million ED visits resulting from sports injuries occur in the pediatric population (4).

The use of nonsteroidal anti-inflammatory drugs (NSAIDs) for pain from musculoskeletal injuries is well known and extensive (3). Musculoskeletal injuries include injuries to muscle, ligaments, tendons, and non-fracture injuries. Treatment of such injuries is generally geared toward reducing the swelling and pain by using methods such as cold compression and an anti-inflammatory agent (5). Typically, the use of NSAIDs is due to their anti-inflammatory, analgesic, and anti-pyretic properties. The basis of the pharmacological action of NSAIDs is their ability to inhibit cylooxygenase (COX) enzymes thereby blocking the formation of certain prostaglandins (PGs). Besides reducing the inflammation, this inhibition of PG synthesis may potentially result in serious side effects such as gastrointestinal disturbance and altered renal function (3,6). Cyclooxygenase-2 (COX-2) inhibitors such as Rofecoxib (Vioxx™) were popular analgesics especially in the last decade. This was because they do not inhibit the beneficial effects of PG's, and thus have fewer side effects on the gastric mucosal lining. They also do not affect bleeding time and platelet function (6). Because of serious cardiovascular side effects reported with the use of COX-2 inhibitors, some of these products were withdrawn from the US markets in 2004 (7).

Due to non-availability of topical form of analgesics in the US market, and because of the negative side effects from a systemic non-steroidal anti-inflammatory drug, an alternative delivery method such as topical can be utilized. A topical route of NSAIDs has the benefit of superior local drug delivery. At the same time the systemic side effects that may arise from oral NSAIDs are reduced by using the topical route (5). A sufficiently high concentration of the drug is necessary to penetrate the skin, muscles, and synovial fluid and this is seen when an NSAID is topically administered. In addition to this benefit, the topical form also allows a constant and slow release of the drug (5).

Review

Literature search was conducted using PubMed and included terms such as "topical NSAIDs", "oral NSAIDs", "sports injuries", "musculoskeletal injuries", and "pain management." Through the synopsis of articles below, this review attempts to emphasize the effectiveness of NSAIDs on pain from acute musculoskeletal sports injuries. It also addresses the use of a topical route as an effective and safe method for NSAID delivery.

* Correspondence: Assistant professor Amit M Deokar, MD, MPH, Department of Pediatrics, Division of Adolescent Medicine (J422), University of Kentucky, Lexington, KY 40536 United States. E-mail: amit-deokar@uky.edu

Discussion

Sports-related injuries that involve the ligaments, muscle, tendons, and bones are fairly common in sports activities. Some studies indicate that there has been a considerable increase in such injuries due to an increased involvement in sports activities (1,4).

Non-steroidal anti-inflammatory drugs are used frequently in pain management of musculoskeletal sports injuries (5). In a randomized controlled trial (RCT) done in an ED setting on patients 6-17 years, who had sustained a musculoskeletal sports injury, an oral non-steroidal, Ibuprofen, was compared with Acetaminophen and Codeine (8). Patients in the Ibuprofen group showed significant improvement compared to the other two groups, as demonstrated on the Visual Analog Scale (VAS). There was twice as much decrease in pain (24mm versus 12mm or 11 mm) on this scale ($p<0.001$). The effectiveness of NSAIDs is due to their mechanism of action that causes inhibition of prostaglandins at the injury site. Oral NSAIDs, when administered in such a situation achieve a relatively higher drug level systemically (3,6). Although this may result in relief of pain symptoms, it may potentially lead to serious side effects such those on gastro protection and renal function. They may also interfere with coagulation mechanisms (9).

There are various routes by which NSAIDs can be delivered. One option is to use the topical route. Topical NSAID's when applied to an inflamed area results in local drug delivery and fewer systemic side effects from high plasma drug levels. One multicenter controlled clinical trial published in the year 2000 compared the effectiveness of the topical Diclofenac Sodium patch to a placebo in patients who had sustained a sports-related injury. Out of the two weeks of treatment, the daily pain relief on days 3, 7, and 14 was superior in the Diclofenac group ($p=0.044$). Another double blinded RCT conducted in Europe compared the Diclofenac patch to a placebo patch, reported significant ($p<0.0001$) pain relief in adult patients who sustained an acute impact sports injury and those who received the active drug (5). This study also reaffirmed the safety and reduced systemic side effects from use of a topical form of an NSAID. Local side effects such as rash or itch occurred similarly in both active as well as inactive patch (5). Another study (randomized double blinded, placebo-controlled) conducted in Europe concluded the efficacy of topical Ketoprofen compared to a placebo in patients who had a benign ankle sprain. This topical NSAID was also tolerated well, with only local side effects (10). Recently, a prospective, randomized, open study compared two topical agents, Ketoprofen and Diclofenac gel in patients who sustained an acute, benign, sports-related injury. The efficacy of transdermal (TDS) Ketoprofen in relieving pain was comparable to the Diclofenac gel. The TDS Ketoprofen was found to be superior to the Diclofenac gel (64% versus 46%, $p=0.004$) leading to a high cure rate on day 7 of the treatment (11). Despite growing evidence that supports the effectiveness of topical NSAID's in pain relief and minimizing the systemic adverse events, several limitations exist for the type of studies conducted thus far in this area. For example, the randomized controlled clinical trials have compared a placebo over a topical form of NSAID to examine the effectiveness and safety profile. While placebo controlled studies are usually preferred to compare the effectiveness of a new drug, it may affect the standard of care for some of the patients. In addition, not many studies have been done exclusively in the pediatric population. Data from the studies done in adults may help researchers conduct clinical trials in children. Topical Diclofenac Sodium formulation is available for use in Europe and other countries (5). In the United States, Dicofenac is available as an oral as well as a topical form. The topical application is a 3% gel that was FDA-approved for Actinic Keratosis in 2002. As of October 2007, the topical Diclofenac Sodium patch was in its Phase 1 clinical study, which is being conducted by Cerimon Pharmaceuticals (12). Numerous clinical trials in the United States are currently undergoing that are looking at the use of topical NSAID for breast pain and osteoarthritis (13). The efficacy of topical non-steroidal anti-inflammatory drugs over a placebo has been noted in various trials involving acute sprain injury as well as chronic conditions such as rheumatoid arthritis (14). Once approved, the topical form of anti-inflammatory drugs is likely to revolutionize the standard of care in pain management of acute benign sports-related musculoskeletal injuries. The use of topical non-steroidal drugs for chronic pain will also be of particular advantage in the elderly population due to their safety profile (14).

References

[1] www.cdc.gov. MMWR Weekly. Sports-Related Injuries Among High School Athletes-United States, 2005-06 School Year. September 29, 2006/55 (38); 1037-1040. Available from: http://www.cdc.gov/mmwr/preview/mmwrhtml/mm5538a1.htm Accessed on 10/08/07.

[2] www.cdc.gov. National Health Interview Survey. National Center for Health Statistics. NCHS-NHIS-Description. Available from: http://cdc.gov/nchs/about/major/nhis/hisdesc.htm Accessd on 10/22/07

[3] Stovitz S, Johnson R. NSAIDs and musculoskeletal treatment. What is the clinical evidence? Physician Sportsmed 2003;31(1). Available from: http://www.chiro.org Accessed on 09/10/07

[4] Tamara S, Bublitz C, Hambridge S. Emergency department visits among pediatric patients for sports-related injury: Basic epidemiology and impact of race/ethnicity and insurance status. Pediatr Emerg Care 2006;22(5):309-15.

[5] Predel HG, Pabst H, Dieter P, Gallacchi G, Giannetti B, Bulitta M, Heidecker J, Mueller E. Diclofenac patch for topical treatment of acute impact injuries: a randomised, double blind, placebo controlled multicenter study. Br J Sports Med 2004;38:318-23.

[6] Paoloni J, Orchard J. The use of therapeutic medications for soft-tissue injuries in sports medicine. Med J Aust 2005;183(7):384-8.

[7] www.fda.gov. Vioxx (rofecoxib) Questions and Answers. 2004. U.S. Food and Drug Administration, Center for Drug Evaluation and Research. Available from: http://www.fda.gov/cder/drug/infopage /vioxx/vioxxQA.htm Accessed on 10/22/07

[8] Clark E, Plint A, Correll R, Gaboury I, Passi B. A randomized controlled trial of acetaminophen, ibuprofen, and codeine for acute pain Relief in children with musculoskeletal trauma. Pediatrics 2007; 119(3): 460-7.

[9] Galer B, Rowotham M, Perander J, Devers A, Friedman E. Topical diclofenac patch relieves minor sports injury pain: Results of a multicenter controlled clinical trial. J Pain Sympt Manage 2000; 19(4):287-94.

[10] Mazieres B, Rouanet S, Velicy J, Scarsi C, Reiner V. Topical ketoprofen (100 mg) for the treatment of ankle sprian: A randomized, double-blind, placebo-controlled study. Am J Sports Med 2005;33(4):515-23.

[11] Esparza F, Cobain C, Jimenez J F, Garcia-Cota Juan, Sanchez C, Maestro A. Topical ketoprofen TDS patch versus diclofenac gel: efficacy and tolerability in benign sport related soft-tissue injuries. Br J Sports Med 2007;41:134-9.

[12] www.cerimon.com. Cerimon Pharmaceuticals. Press Release, October 2007. Available from: http://www.cerimon.com/news/041007.html Accessed on 10/22/07

[13] www.clinicaltrials.gov. Trial list. Search: Diclofenac Sodium. Available from: ttp://www.clinicaltrials gov/ct/search;jsessionid=9343FACF0E0E3BF3AC011DA0522316DA?term=diclofenac+sodium+and submit=Search Accessed on 10/22/07

[14] Moore R, Tramer M, Carroll D, Wiffen P, McQuay H. Quantitive systematic review of topically applied non-steroidal anti-inflammatory drugs. BMJ 1998;316:333-8.

In: Children and Pain
Editors: P. Schofield and J. Merrick
ISBN 978-1-60876-020-6

Chapter 4

Treatment during acute painful episodes in adolescents with sickle cell disease

***Eufemia Jacob, PhD, RN*[*1], *Marilyn Hockenberry, PhD, RN-CS, PNP, FAAN*[2,3] *and Brigitta U Mueller, MD, MHCM*[4,5]**
[1]UCLA School of Nursing, Los Angeles, California
[2]Department of Hematology/Oncology, Baylor College of Medicine
[3]Center for Research and Evidence-Based Practice,
Texas Children's Hospital, Houston, Texas
[4]Division of Clinical Services, Texas Children's Cancer Center
[5]Hematology Service, Texas Children's Sickle Cell Center,
Baylor College of Medicine, Houston, Texas, USA

Abstract

The use of hydromorphone is increasing but little is known about its effects during painful episodes in children and adolescents with sickle cell disease. This pilot study examined the intensity, location, and quality of pain and evaluated the amount of relief and side effects from PCA hydromorphone during acute painful episodes in five adolescents with sickle cell disease.

Data suggest that hydromorphone may provide a better alternative than morphine, the most commonly prescribed opioid in patients with sickle cell disease. Hydromorphone may provide improved pain control and recovery from acute painful episodes in patients with sickle cell disease.

---

[*] Correspondence: Assistant professor Eufemia Jacob, PhD, RN, UCLA School of Nursing, Factor Building 5-942, 700 Tiverton Avenue, Los Angeles, CA 90095-6919, United States. Tel: (310) 267-1823; Fax: (310) 206-3241; E-mail: ejacob@sonnet.ucla.edu

Introduction

The acute painful episode is the hallmark of sickle cell disease and accounts for the most frequent reason for emergency department visits and hospitalization in these patients (1,2). The mainstay of pain therapy is treatment of the underlying cause, rest, hydration and opioids, predominantly morphine (3). The use of hydromorphone is increasing (4), particularly for patients who are experiencing untolerable itching, increased sedation, or unresponsive to and requiring high doses of morphine (clinical experience). However, data on the effects of hydromorphone on pain intensity ratings, pain location, and pain quality are lacking in children and adolescents with sickle cell disease.

Hydromorphone may be more preferrable over morphine because of its solubility and speed of onset (5,6). Patients also report few troublesome side effects. Furthermore, hydromorphone has lower dependence liability as compared to morphine. As part of a larger study that examined analgesic response to morphine in patients with sickle cell disease, we examined the intensity, location, and quality of pain in patients receiving hydromorphone. The specific aims of this report are: 1) to examine the intensity, location, and quality of pain and 2) to evaluate the amount of relief and side effects from PCA hydromorphone during acute painful episodes in adolescents with sickle cell disease.

A pilot study

The data presented here were part of a study that examined the effects of different PCA regimens in children and adolescents with sickle cell disease during hospitalization for acute painful episodes. Patients with sickle cell disease were recruited from the hematology unit of a large children's hospital in the central southern United States. The Sickle Cell Program in this facility follows about 900 patients per year and provides comprehensive services for patients with sickle cell disease.

All hospitalized patients with sickle cell disease, eight years and older, were eligible. The age of eight years was chosen as the cut-off point because the outcome measures for pain were validated for patients eight years and older. In addition, patients younger than eight years old were less likely prescribed patient controlled analgesia for pain management during acute painful episodes. Patients were included in the study if: 1) they were English-speaking (data collection instruments available only in English); 2) the primary reason for admission was for management of acute pain as documented by the attending physician in the admission records, and 3) the pain was severe enough to require the administration of intravenous PCA opioids. Patients with sickle cell disease were excluded if pain was not related to an acute painful episode (infection, surgery, burns, trauma). Patients were also excluded if they had cognitive and neurological impairments that precluded them from completing the pain tool. The study was approved by the Institutional Review Board of the medical center.

Procedures

Children were asked to rate pain using 0 to 10 numerical rating scales (0=no pain to 10=a lot of pain) for 1) worst pain, 2) least pain, and 3) amount of pain relief during treatment (0=no relief to 10=complete relief). The 0 to 10 numeric rating scale is a well-established valid and reliable tool (14), and was previously used by children with sickle cell disease (7-8). A checklist that consisted of common side effects of morphine (hypotension, bradycardia, respiratory depression, drowsiness, dizziness, tremors, sedation, pruritus, nausea, vomiting, constipation, urinary retention) was used to record side effects.

The patient was also asked to complete the Adolescent Pediatric Pain Tool (APPT) to measure the intensity, location, and quality of pain. Reliability and validity of the APPT is well established (9-13). Previous APPT data from children with sickle cell disease showed that pain location and spatial distribution of pain changed during acute painful episodes even when pain intensity remained the same (14).

The patient's Medication Administration Record was reviewed for the dose, route, and time of all medications that were administered for pain (e.g. nonsteroidal anti-inflammatory drugs [NSAIDs] such as ibuprofen and ketorolac) and for side effects (e.g., diphenhydramine for itching, hydroxyzine and odansetron for emesis). In addition, the following information were also collected from the medical records: 1) demographic information such as age, gender, weight, height, hemoglobin genotype; and 2) health related information such as CBC, pain ratings in the ED, presence of fever, oxygen saturation, other signs and symptoms at time of admission, history of past complications and sickle cell related treatments.

Data analyses

Scatter plots were used to describe worst and least pain patterns across the five days. Descriptive statistics (frequencies, means, standard deviations) were used to describe worst and least pain, location of pain, and quality of pain, type and amount of medications, and amount of relief.

Results

The patients who were prescribed PCA hydromorphone had a mean age of 16.2 ± 2.5 years, mostly female (4F; 1M), and had predominantly HgBSS genotype. In the ED, they received a morphine equivalent (0.07 mg/kg/dose) of hydromorphone. The least pain was 2.7 ± 1.1 and the worst pain was 8.5 ± 1.3. The onset of pain was 2 ± 1.2 days prior to admission. The mean length of stay was 6.4 ± 4.4 days.

The recommended hydromorphone PCA dosing schedule as recommended by the American Pain Society (15) is presented in table 1. Patients self-administered 15 to 20 mg of hydromorphone/day (morphine equivalent to 0.3 mg/kg/day; see example of patient daily consumption of hydromorphone, table 1).

Table 1. Hydromorphone Patient Controlled Analgesia Regimen

**Recommendation for Patient Controlled Analgesia Settings (PCA) Hydromorphone		Example PCA Settings for 60 kg Patient
Loading Dose	20 microgram/kg (max 1.5 mg)	1300 mcg (1.3 mg)
Intermittent Push	5 microgram/kg/dose	300 mcg (0.3 mg/dose)
Background Rate	1.5 microgram/kg/hour	90 mcg (0.09 mg/hour)
Lock-out Interval	6 to 8 minutes	6 to 8 minutes
4 hour Maximum	20 microgram/kg/hour	4800 mcg (4.8 mg)

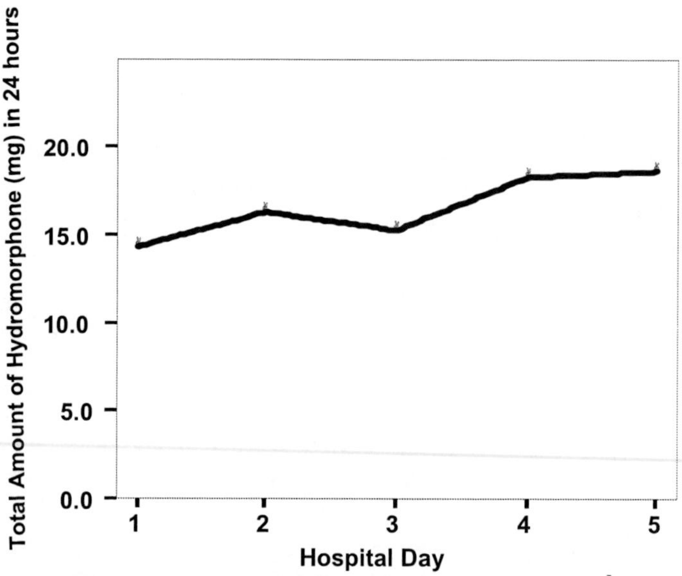

mcg: micrograms; mg: milligrams.

**Recommended Dosing Schedule from: Benjamin LJ, Dampier CD, Jacox aK, Odesina V, Phoenix D, Shapiro B, Strafford M, Treadwell M: Guideline for the Management of Acute and Chronic Pain in Sickle Cell Disease. Glenview,IL, American Pain Society, 1999; Taketomo, C. K., Hodding, J. H., & Kraus, D. M. Pediatric Dosage Handbook. Hudson, Ohio: Lexi-comp, Inc. 2007.

The trends in worst (range 5.7 to 9.0 on 0 to 10 NRS) and least (range 2.5 to 5.5 on 0 to 10 NRS) pain intensity ratings during the course of hospitalization are illustrated in figure 1. The number of body areas marked with pain ranged from 5.8 to 9 areas (figure 2A). The number of quality word descriptors selected ranged from 5.3 to 17 (figure 2B). The most frequent words were sensory quality (2.0 to 6.4), and fewer affective (0.5 to 2.8), evaluative (1.5 to 5.8), and temporal words (1.0 to 4.0). The perceived amount of pain relief (4.2 to 5.5 on 0 to 10 NRS) during the course of hospitalization is illustrated in figure 3.

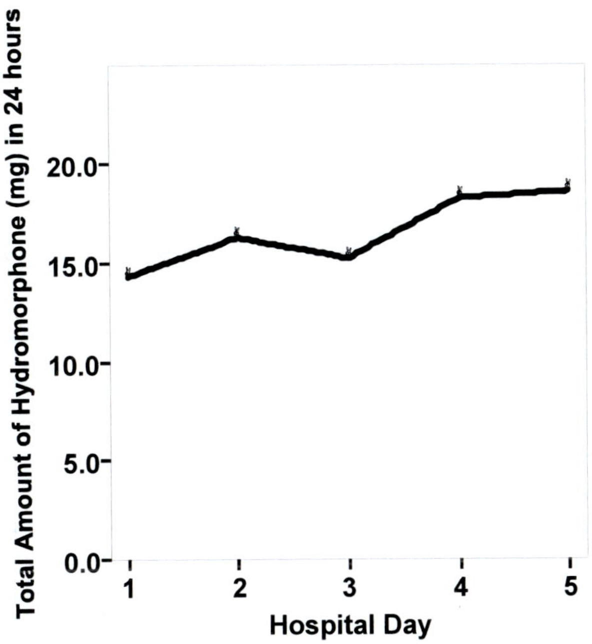

Example of Daily Hydromorphone Consumption for 60 kg Patient.

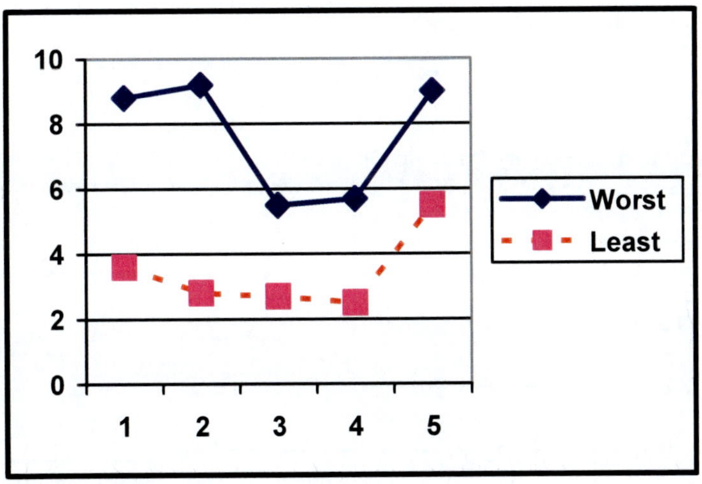

Figure 1. Worst and Least Pain Intensity Ratings on 0 to 10 NRS.

Itching was the most common side effect, reported by 4 of the 5 patients in the PCA hydromorphone regimen. Nausea and vomiting were reported by one patient. No one had low blood pressure, heart rate, or respiratory rate. One patient had difficulty stooling, which was reported prior to enrollment.

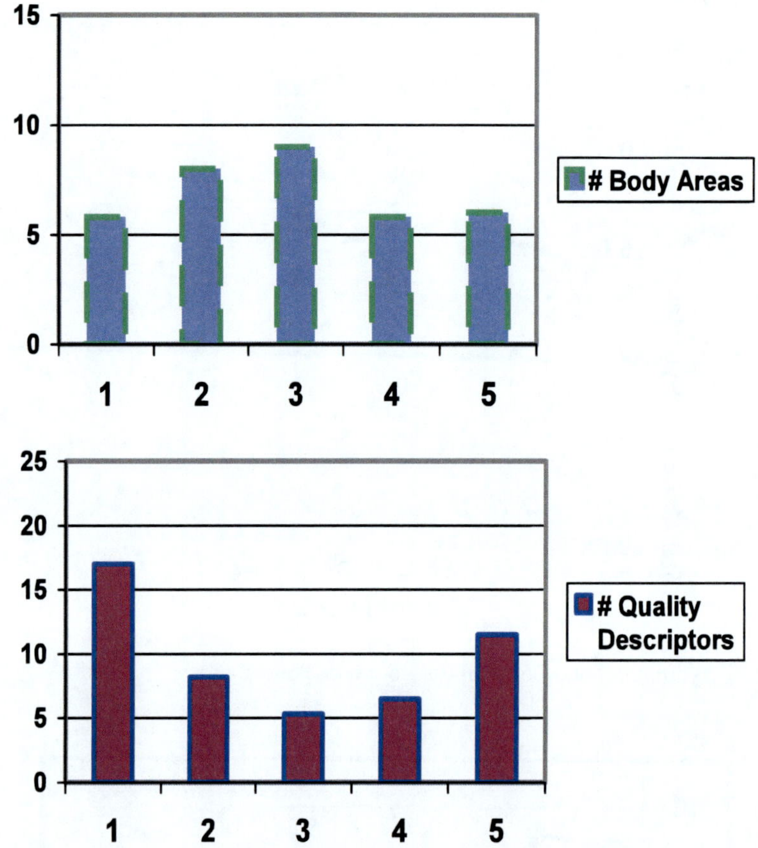

Figure 2. Number of Body Areas Marked on the Body Outline Diagram (A) and Number of Quality Descriptors (B) Selected to Descript Pain in Adolescents with Sickle Cell Disease.

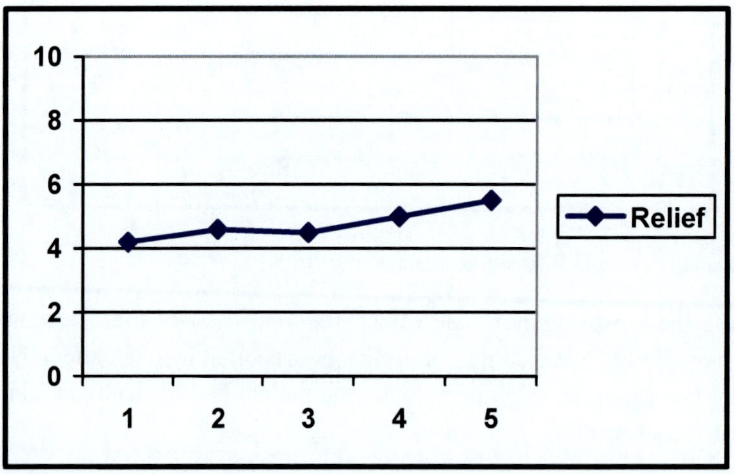

Figure 3. Amount of Relief on 0 to 10 NRS.

Conclusions

While previous reports have examined the effects of morphine on the intensity, location, and quality of pain in children with sickle cell disease (7,8,14), very little if any reports were available that examined the effects of hydromorphone during acute painful episodes.

We found that pain intensity ratings decreased over time with PCA hydromorphone in this small sample of adolescents. We observed that with PCA hydromorphone, worst pain decreased by at least 20% (figure 1). Furthermore, our data showed that least pain intensity ratings were lower during the course of hospitalization than were reported in previous studies (7,8,14). Jacob and colleagues reported that patients with sickle cell disease showed that morphine decreased pain intensity ratings by 5% (14) which was not clinically significant. However, because our sample size was small for both the hydromorphone and morphine, we were not able to make any statistical analyses to tests for significance.

The number of body areas marked with pain was not affected by the use of hydromorphone. However, the number of word descriptors to describe the quality of pain showed a decreasing trend. The amount of pain relief from hydromorphone remained moderate throughout hospitalization. Very few patients reported side effects (itching, nausea, vomiting).

Although this study represented a small number of patients with sickle cell disease and would not be representative of the experience of all patients with acute painful episodes, our data suggest that hydromorphone may provide a better alternative than morphine, which is the most commonly prescribed opioid in patients with sickle cell disease (7,8). Therefore, we recommend future studies to examine whether hydromorphone is more effective in improving pain and recovery from acute painful episodes in children with sickle cell disease. A report by Perlman and colleagues (4) showed that hydromorphone improved pain control and decreased admissions for acute painful episodes in adult patients with sickle cell disease.

Acknowledgments

Funding from this study is provided by a Mentored Patient-Oriented Research Career Development Award (#5K23NR009192) from the National Institute of Nursing Research.

References

[1] Ballas SK, Lusardi M. Hospital readmission for adult acute sickle cell painful episodes: frequency, etiology, and prognostic significance. Am J Hematol 2005;79:17–25.

[2] Platt OS, Thorington BD, Brambilla DJ et al. Pain in sickle cell disease. Rates and risk factors. N Engl J Med 1991;325:11–6.

[3] Ellison AM, Shaw K. Management of vasoocclusive pain events in sickle cell disease. Pediatr Emerg Care 2007;23(11):832-8.

[4] Perlman KM, Myers-Phariss S, Rhodes JC. A shift from demerol (Meperidine) to dilaudid (Hydromorphone) improves pain control and decreases admissions for patients in sickle cell crisis. J Emerg Nurs 2004;30(5):439-46.

[5] Taketomo CK, Hodding JH, Kraus DM. Pediatric dosage handbook. Hudson, Ohio: Lexi-comp, 2007.

[6] Brunton L, Lazo J, Lazo, JS. Goodman and Gilman's pharmacological basis of therapeutics, 11th ed. New York: McGraw-Hill, 2005;569-620.

[7] Jacob E, Miaskowski C, Savedra M, Beyer JE, Treadwell M, Styles L. Management of vaso-occlusive pain in hospitalized children with sickle cell disease. J Pediatr Hematol Oncol 2003;25(4):307-11.

[8] Jacob E, Mueller B. Pain and symptom experience in hospitalized children with sickle cell disease who had prolonged hospitalizations. Pain Med 1Feb 2007. [Epub ahead of print]

[9] Savedra M, Tesler M, Holzemer WL, Wilkie DJ, Ward JA. Testing a tool to assess postoperative pediatric and adolescent pain. In: Tyler DC, Krane EJ, eds. Advances in pain research and therapy: Pediatric pain. New York: Raven Press, 1990;15.

[10] Savedra MC, Holzemer WL, Tesler MD, Wilkie DJ. Assessment of postoperation pain in children and adolescents. Using the adolescent pediatric pain tool. Nurs Res 1993;42(1):5-9.

[11] Savedra MC, Tesler MD, Holzemer WL, Wilkie DJ, Ward JA. Pain location: Validity and reliability of body outline markings by hospitalized children and adolescents. Res Nurs Health 1989;12: 307-14.

[12] Wilkie DJ, Holzemer WL, Tesler MD, Ward JA, Paul SM, Savedra MC. Measuring pain quality: Validity and reliability of children's and adolescents' pain language. Pain 1990;41:151-9.

[13] Franck LS, Treadwell M, Jacob E, Vichinsky E. Assessment of sickle cell pain in children and young adults using the adolescent pediatric pain tool. J Pain Sympt Manage 2002;23:114-20.

[14] Jacob E, Miaskowski C, Savedra M, Beyer JE, Treadwell M, Styles L. Changes in intensity, location, and quality of vaso-occlusive pain. Pain 2003;102(1-2):187-93.

[15] Benjamin LJ, Dampier CD, Jacox AK, Odesina V, Phoenix D, Shapiro B, Strafford M, Treadwell M. Guideline for the management of acute and chronic pain in sickle cell disease. Glenview, IL: Am Pain Society, 1999.

In: Children and Pain
Editors: P. Schofield and J. Merrick
ISBN 978-1-60876-020-6

Chapter 5

Morphine for acute pain in children with sickle cell disease

***Eufemia Jacob, PhD, RN*[*1], *Marilyn Hockenberry, PhD, RN-CS, PNP, FAAN*[2,3], *Brigitta U Mueller, MD, MHCM*[4,5], *Thomas D Coates, MD*[6] *and Lonnie Zeltzer, MD*[7,8,9]**
[1]UCLA School of Nursing, Los Angeles, California
[2]Departtment of Hematology/Oncology, Baylor College of Medicine
[3]Center for Research and Evidence-Based Practice,
Texas Children's Hospital, Houston, Texas
[4]Division of Clinical Services,
Texas Children's Cancer Center and Hematology Service,
Baylor College of Medicine, Houston, Texas
[5]Texas Children's Sickle Cell Center, Houston, Texas
[6]Sickle Cell/Hemoglobinopathy Program,
Childrens Center for Cancer and Blood Diseases, Los Angeles, California
[7]David Geffen School of Medicine at UCLA
[8]Pediatric Pain Program, UCLA Mattel Children's Hospital and Patients
[9]Survivors Program, UCLA Jonsson Cancer Center, Los Angeles,
California, United States of America

Abstract

Morphine given by Patient Controlled Analgesia (PCA) is widely used in hospital settings to manage severe pain during acute painful episodes. Wide variations in prescription patterns occur and some patients are often self-administering sub- or low-therapeutic doses. In this preliminary study, a descriptive design with repeated measures was used to examine the effects of different PCA morphine regimens on the intensity,

[*] Correspondence: Assistant professor Eufemia Jacob, PhD, RN, UCLA School of Nursing, Factor Building 5-942, 700 Tiverton Avenue, Los Angeles, CA 90095-6919, United States. Tel: (310) 267-1823; Fax: (310) 206-3241; E-mail: ejacob@sonnet.ucla.edu

location and quality of pain as well as on the perceived amount of relief and side effects in patients with sickle cell disease (N=13; mean age 13.7 years; eight males; five females). The preliminary data showed that a regimen with a high background infusion rate and low intermittent push dose (Regimen B) may provide better response to PCA morphine. The difference in trends between the worst and least pain intensity ratings were narrower in this regimen, suggesting that pain peaks and troughs were not occurring as in a regimen with an around the clock nurse administered dosing schedule (Regimen C). The amount of morphine that was administered per day was not significantly different ($p > 0.05$) among the three morphine regimens. The combination of a high background infusion rate and low intermittent push dose (as in Regimen B) within the first 24 hours of admission, may provide improved response and possibly shorter recovery from the painful episode than the regimen that would routinely be prescribed with lower background infusion rate and high intermittent push dose (as in regimen A).

Introduction

Sickle cell disease is an inherited disorder that affects one in 500 African Americans (1,2). The acute painful episode is the most common problem in children with sickle cell disease. It may be a manifestation of vaso-occlusion or may be a symptom of another process, such as infection. The painful episode due to vaso-occlusion is the most frequent cause for emergency department visits and hospital admissions (3,4).

Painful episodes that are severe enough to require hospitalization typically last 3 to 7 days, but pain may persist for as long as several weeks (5). Children may experience persistent pain of mild to moderate intensity on a daily basis, or may have intermittent acute exacerbations of more severe pain. In most cases during the acute painful episode, pain intensity increases rapidly, plateaus, and then falls, but the pattern may be unpredictable (6,7). Morphine given by PCA is widely used in hospital settings to manage severe pain during acute painful episodes (8-10). However, there were wide variations in prescription patterns, and patients were often self-administering sub- or low-therapeutic doses, commonly 35% on the average of what were prescribed. The most common PCA morphine regimen consisted of high intermittent push dose and low background infusion rate (8-10). With this PCA morphine regimen, children were most likely falling asleep in between the intermittent push doses and waking up with pain, and leading to a "prn" dosing schedule and thus, not providing optimal relief. Therefore, pain intensity ratings remained at moderate to high levels through the course of hospitalization (8,9) and some patients with sickle cell disease had prolonged hospitalizations associated with persistent pain (10).

It is not known if other combinations of PCA settings, such as increasing the background infusion, or having larger amounts administered around the clock (ATC) may provide better response to morphine. Such regimens could achieve a more steady concentration of the drug associated with the "ATC" dosing schedule, rather than a "PRN" dosing schedule with peaks and troughs (11,12). Therefore, the purpose of this preliminary study was to examine the effects of the different PCA regimens on the intensity, location and quality of pain as well as on the perceived amount of relief and side effects.

Our study

A descriptive design with repeated measures was used to examine the effects of the different PCA regimens during hospitalization for acute painful episodes. Patients with sickle cell disease were recruited from the hematology unit of a large children's hospital in the central southern United States. The Sickle Cell Program in this facility follows about 900 patients per year and provides comprehensive services for patients with sickle cell disease.

Inclusion criteria

All hospitalized patients with sickle cell disease, eight years and older, were eligible. The age of eight years was chosen as the cut-off point because the outcome measures for pain were validated for patients eight years and older. In addition, patients younger than 8 years old were less likely prescribed patient controlled analgesia for pain management during acute painful episodes. Patients were included in the study if: 1) they were English-speaking (data collection instruments available only in English); 2) the primary reason for admission was for management of acute pain as documented by the attending physician in the admission records, and 3) the pain was severe enough to require the administration of intravenous morphine.

Exclusion criteria

Patients with sickle cell disease were excluded if pain was not related to an acute painful episode (infection, surgery, burns, trauma). Patients were also excluded if they had cognitive and neurological impairments that precluded them from completing the pain tool. They were excluded if they were already receiving morphine at doses above the study entry dose (either an intermittent push dose setting greater than 0.07 mg/dose, a background infusion rate setting greater than 0.03 mg/kg/hr, or a four hour limit setting greater than 0.6 mg/kg (equivalent to 0.15 mg/kg one hour limit setting) . The decision to exclude patients was made by the PI in consultation with the hematology team. The study was approved by the Institutional Review Board of the medical center.

Procedures

Patients were randomly assigned to one of three morphine regimens (Regimen A, B, or C). The differences among the regimens were in the combination of settings programmed in the PCA device. The settings differed in: 1) the amount given by background infusion, 2) the amount given by the intermittent push button, and 3) the lockout interval settings programmed in the PCA device (see table 1). The 4 hour maximum [converted to hourly equivalent] setting prescribed for each regimen was controlled to minimize the confounding effect of dose on the variation in response. The hourly limit setting was standardized in mg/kg/hour based on the amount that is recommended in the Pediatric Drug Dosage Handbook (13), a medication reference book which is widely used in children's hospitals as part of the formulary across the United States.

Table 1. Morphine patient controlled analgesia regimens

	Patient Controlled Analgesia Morphine Regimens		
	A (N=5)	B (N=5)	C (N=3)
Intermittent Push	0.07 mg/kg/dose	0.035 mg/kg/dose	0.15 mg/kg/dose
Background Rate	0.015 mg/kg/hr	0.03 mg/kg/hr	0.00 mg/kg/hr
Lock-out Interval	10 minutes	10 minutes	180 minutes [q 3 hrs]
4 hour Maximum [Hourly Maximum]	0.6 mg/kg [0.15 mg/kg/hr]	0.6 mg/kg [0.15 mg/kg/hr]	0.6 mg/kg
Example PCA Settings for a 40 kg patient for the different regimens:			
	Patient Controlled Analgesia Morphine Regimens		
	A	B	C
Intermittent Push	2.8 mg	1.4 mg	6 mg
Background Rate	0.6 mg/kg/hr	1.2 mg	0.0 mg/kg/hr
Lock-out Interval	10 minutes	10 minutes	180 minutes [q 3 hrs]
4 hour Maximum [Hourly Maximum]	24 mg [6 mg/kg/hr]	24 mg [6 mg/kg/hr]	

Patient controlled analgesia morphine regimens

Patients in Regimen A were prescribed the regimen of higher intermittent push (HIP) dose (0.07 mg/kg/dose; proportionally two times the intermittent push dose prescribed for regimen B) and lower background infusion (LBI) rate (0.015 mg/kg/hr; proportionately half the amount prescribed for regimen B). The maximum 4-hour limit setting for this regimen was 0.6 mg/kg, equivalent to 0.15 mg/kg/hr x 4 hours (9,10). The recommended therapeutic dose range from the Pediatric Drug Dosage Handbook commonly used by children's hospitals across the country is 0.1 to 0.2 mg/kg/hr (13); thus the hourly dose selected for this study is in the midpoint of the therapeutic dose range.

Patients in regimen B were prescribed the opposite regimen of lower intermittent push (LIP) dose (0.03 mg/kg/dose; proportionally half from Regimen A) and higher background infusion (HBI) rate regimen (0.03 mg/kg/hr; proportionately two times the background rate in Regimen A). The 4-hour maximum limit setting for this regimen was also 0.6 mg/kg [0.15

mg/kg/hr x 4 hours], which was the same as the maximum 4-hour limiting setting for regimen A (13). Thus, the hourly limit setting was standardized for the morphine PCA regimens in the study.

Patients in regimen C [Nurse Controlled Analgesia] were prescribed an around the clock (ATC) dose of 0.15 mg/kg/dose, based on the recommended parameters of 0.1 to 0.2 mg/kg/dose every 3 hours; maximum 15 mg/dose (13). This dose was higher than the dose that could be delivered by PCA in a background infusion rate or in an intermittent push dose, but equivalent to the dose that would be prescribed if PCA was not available. However, for this study, regimen C was delivered using the PCA device with the intermittent push dose rate setting at 0.15 mg/kg/dose and background infusion rate set at 0.0; lockout interval was set at 180 minutes (three hours) to allow the nurse to push the dose every three hours, and simulate a “q 3 hour ATC” regimen, that was typically prescribed for patients without using the PCA device. Thus, no intermittent dose for patient to push and no background infusion rate were prescribed for Regimen C. In general, medications administered ATC achieve stead state levels after 4 to 5 half-lifes (half-life of morphine is two hours) (14). Therefore, even though this regimen was administered intermittently every three hours ATC, the level of mophine in the blood is expected to reach steady state after two to three doses, a level that would be achieved if patient had a background infusion rate.

All patients were enrolled within 48 hours of initiation of PCA and they were prescribed the study dose for 24 hours. In the event that the patient required additional doses beyond the assigned study settings, a PRN dose was prescribed for all regimens at 0.05 mg/kg/dose (33% of the one hour limit study setting, i.e. 0.05 mg/kg/hr). This amount was based on the rescue dose recommended by the American Pain Society Guideline for the Management of Acute and Chronic Sickle Cell Disease, which is recommended at 25% to 50% of the hourly opioid dose (15). If the patient required three additional doses in any one hour period beyond the study PCA settings before hour 24, the physician could change the PCA settings and the patient would be off study.

Outcome measures

Children were asked to rate pain using 0 to 10 numerical rating scales (0=no pain to 10=a lot of pain) for 1) worst pain, 2) least pain, and 3) amount of pain relief during treatment (0=no relief to 10=complete relief). The 0 to 10 numeric rating scale is a well-established valid and reliable tool (16), and was previously used by children with sickle cell disease (8-10). A checklist that consisted of common side effects of morphine (hypotension, bradycardia, respiratory depression, drowsiness, dizziness, tremors, sedation, pruritus, nausea, vomiting, constipation, urinary retention) was used to record side effects.

The patient was also asked to complete the Adolescent Pediatric Pain Tool (APPT) to measure the intensity, location, and quality of pain. Reliability and validity of the APPT is well established (17-20). Previous APPT data from children with sickle cell disease showed that pain location and spatial distribution of pain changed during acute painful episodes even when pain intensity remained the same (8).

The patient's Medication Administration Record was reviewed for the dose, route, and time of all medications that were administered for pain (e.g. nonsteroidal anti-inflammatory drugs [NSAIDs] such as ibuprofen and ketorolac) and for side effects (e.g., diphenhydramine for itching, hydroxyzine and odansetron for emesis). In addition, the following information were also collected from the medical records: 1) demographic information such as age, gender, weight, height, hemoglobin genotype; and 2) health related information such as CBC, pain ratings in the ED, presence of fever, oxygen saturation, other signs and symptoms at time of admission, history of past complications and sickle cell related treatments.

Data analyses

Scatter plots were used to describe worst and least pain patterns across the five days. Descriptive statistics (frequencies, means, standard deviations) were used to describe worst and least pain, location of pain, and quality of pain, type and amount of medications, and amount of relief.

Results

During the two year study period between August, 2005 and July, 2007, 326 sickle cell related admissions were screened in the hematology unit, with an average of 18.1 ± 5.6 admissions each month. These admissions represented 160 patients; 30% had three or more repeat admissions. Among the 160 patients, 68 (42.8%) patients were admitted for reasons other than acute painful episodes, 28 (17.6%) patients had acute painful episode, but did not have PCA morphine at time of screening and recruitment, 14 (8.8%) were excluded for various reasons (such as, developmental delay, communication disorder, behavioral problems, disruptive behavior, cognitive dysfunction, neurological impairments, patient not appropriate for randomization, parent noncompliant or not appropriate for consenting procedures, patient on legal custody and parent/legal guardian not known), 8 (5.0%) were weaned from pain medications and were planned to be discharged within 24 hours, 4 (2.5%) were eligible, but enrolled in a concurrent study, 2 (1.3%) did not have parents available for consent, 16 (10.1%) refused. A total of 15 patients were randomized in the PCA morphine regimens; two of them (1 from regimen C; the other from regimen A) had withdrawn early. The 13 patients who completed the study were randomly assigned to Regimen A (n=5), B (n=5), and C (n=5).

Baseline characteristics of patients in regimen A (n=5), B (n=5), and C (n=3) were not significantly different (N=13; mean age 13.7 years; eight males; five females; table 2). The Hemoglobin phenotype was predominantly HgbSS (n=9). Onset of pain was 1.7 to 3.4 days prior to admission. Lowest mean pain intensity ratings in the Emergency Department (ED) prior to admission ranged from 5.0 to 7.7, with the highest pain intensity ratings from 7.3 to 9.5 on 0 to 10 numerical ratings scales (NRS). Patients received 0.08 to 0.10 mg/kg/dose, which were lower or within the lower range of the recommended morphine dose of 0.1 to 0.2

mg/kg/dose (12). Patients in regimen B had an overall mean shorter length of stay (Table 1); however this was not statistically significant (p > 0.05).

Table 2. Demographics

	A (N=5)	B (N=5)	C (N=3)
Age (years)	13.6 ± 2.1 (11 – 17)	13.0 ± 2.0 (10 – 16)	14.7 ± 4.2 (range 10 – 18)
Weight (kg)	49.5 ± 18.3 (31.0 to 76.0)	70.5 ± 18.6 (42.0 to 93.6)	48.1 ± 24.0 (26.5.0 to 74.0)
Height (cm)	158.5 ± 11.9 (145.5 to 169.0)	153.7 ± 20.7 (127.0 to 174.0)	151.1 ± 13.0 (141.0 to 166.0)
Gender			
Male	4	3	1
Female	1	2	2
Hemoglobin			
SS	4	2	3
SC	1	1	--
S Beta	--	1	--
Pain Onset (Number Days PTA)	1.8 ± 1.5 (1 to 4)	1.7 ± 0.6 (1 to 2)	3.4 ± 4.6 (1 to 9)
Lowest Pain in ER (0 to 10 NRS)	7.7 ± 2.1 (6 to 10)	7.0 ± 3.3 (0 to 7)	5.0 ± 1.4 (4 to 6)
Highest Pain in ER (0 to 10 NRS)	9.5 ± 1.0 (8 to 10)	7.3 ± 1.2 (6 to 8)	9.0 ± 1.4 (8 to10)
Morphine in ER (mg/kg/dose)	0.08	0.09	0.10
Length of Hospital Stay (days)	6.0 2.2 3 to 9	5.6 2.4 3 to 9	7.0 2.6 7 to 10

PTA: Prior to Admission; ER: Emergency Room.

Pain intensity

The worst pain intensity ratings in Regimen B decreased significantly during the course of hospitalization (see figure 1). The worst pain intensity rating was 9.5 on day 1 and 5.5 on day 5, p=0.01 for Regimen B. The worst pain intensity ratings for patients on regimen A (9.8 to 9.0, p > 0.05) and regimen C (9.6 to 7.5, p>0.05) did not change significantly during hospitalization (see figure 1). The least pain intensity ratings of patients in regimen C were lower than patients in either regimen A or B (see figure 2). The difference in trends between the worst and least pain intensity ratings across the hospital days was widest in regimen C when compared to either Regimen A or B (see figure 2).

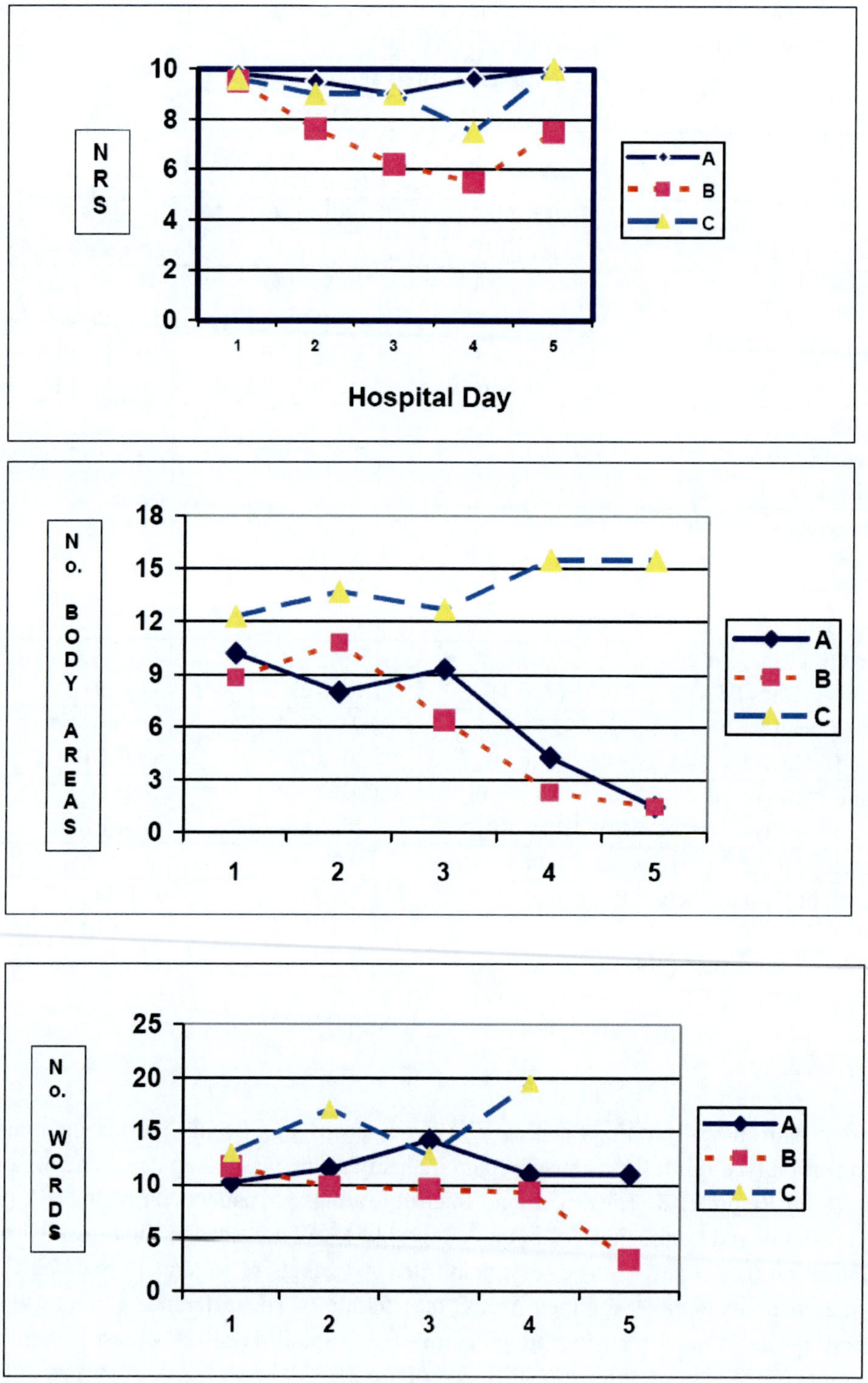

Figure 1. Pain intensity ratings (A), Number of body areas (B) and number of quality word descriptors (C) Day 1 to Day 5 of hospitalization.

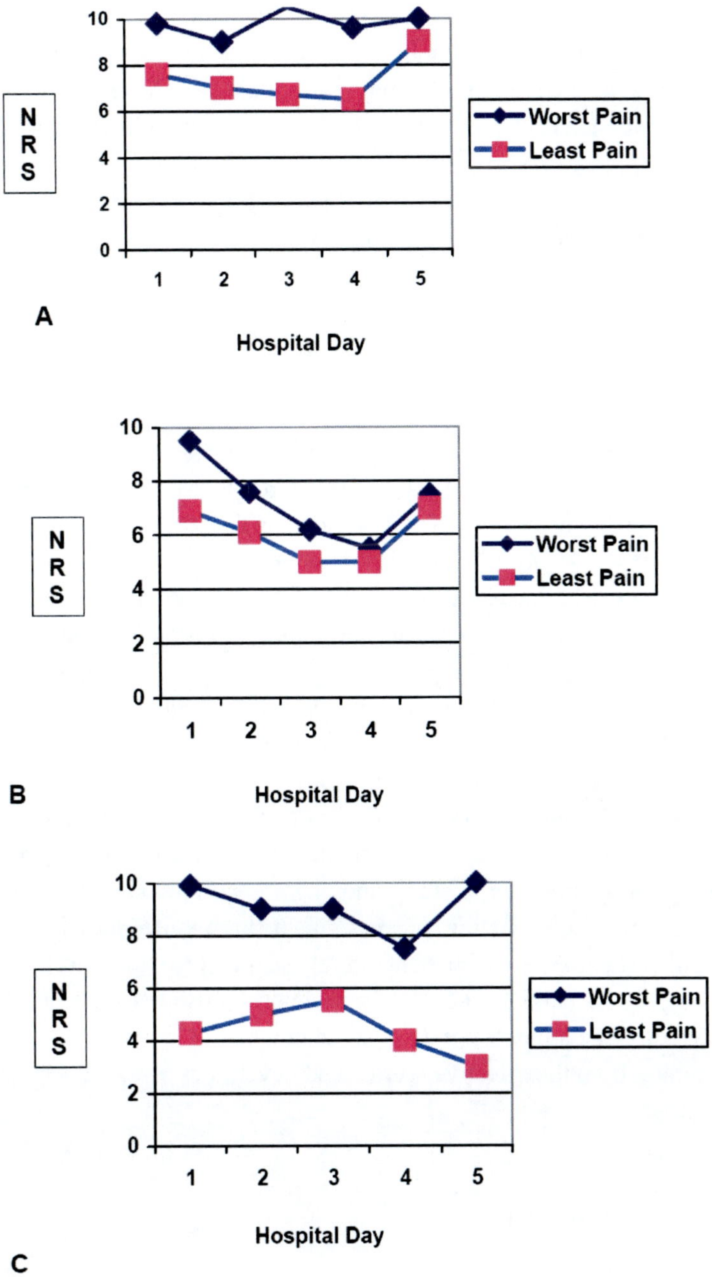

Figure 2. Comparison of worst and least pain ratings for regimen A, B, C.

Pain location

The most frequent areas marked for pain by patients in regimen A were the right upper arm (75%), right abdomen (50%), left thigh and knees (50%), right back chest (50%), and lower back (50%). The most frequent areas marked by patients in Regimen B were chest (83%), right knee (50%), and left thigh and knees (50%). Patients in regimen C marked the chest (66.7%), right upper arm (66.7%), right abdomen (66.7%), and lower back (66.7%).

The number of areas marked on the body outline diagram remained constant throughout hospitalization for regimen C (12.3 to 15.5 areas). The number of areas marked decreased for patients in regimen A (10.2 to 1.5) and B (8.8 to 1.5). Worst pain intensity ratings remained at moderate levels (see figure 1A) throughout hospitalization; however, the number of body areas marked with pain decreased for regimen A and B, but not for regimen C (see figure 1B).

Pain quality

The number of words to describe the quality of pain remained similar throughout hospitalization from 10.2 on day 1 to 11.0 on day 5 ($p > 0.05$) for patients on regimen A (see figure 1C). The most frequent words were sensory quality (3.7 to 7.5), and fewer affective (1.75 to 2.5), evaluative (2.2 to 2.7), or temporal words (1.7 to 2.5). The number of words to describe the quality of pain decreased from 11.7 to 3.0 for patients on regimen B (see figure 1C). The most frequent words were also sensory quality (3.6 to 6.0) and fewer affective (0.8 to 1.3), evaluative (1.7 to 2.2), or temporal words (1.8 to 2.6). For patients in regimen C, the number of words remained similar throughout hospitalization, and slightly increased from 13.0 on day 1 to 19.2 on day 5 ($p>0.05$). The number of sensory (6.3 to 10.0), affective (2.3 to 3.0), evaluative (2.3 to 4.0), and temporal quality words (2.0 to 3.0) were slightly higher, but not significantly different ($p>0.05$) from the patients in regimen A and B.

The words that were selected by 75% of patients in regimen A to describe the quality of pain were hurting, sharp, pressure, awful, annoying and continuous. The majority of patients (66.7%) in regimen B selected aching, hurting, like a sharp knife, shooting, dizzy, annoying, and uncomfortable. The majority of patients in regimen C (66.7%) selected similar words. In addition, the majority of patients (66.7%) in regimen C also selected other words such as throbbing, tight, sore, like a pinch, stinging, shocking, and pounding from the sensory words; crying and sickening from the affective words; and never goes away, steady, and always from the temporal words.

Daily morphine consumption

The amount of morphine that was administered per day was not significantly different ($p>0.05$) among the three regimens (see figure 3A). Patients in regimen A were administered on the average from 59.4 mg on day 1 to 33.8 mg on day 5. This amount was equivalent to 1.2 mg/kg/day on day 1 to 1.1 mg/kg/day on day 5. The largest amount was administered on day 3 (77.3 mg/day or 1.4 mg/kg/day). Patients in regimen B had consistently decreased in the amount of morphine that was administered during hospitalization from 73.5 mg/day on day 1 to 23.5 mg/day on day 5 (equivalent to 1.1 on day 1 to 0.3 mg/kg/day on day 5). Patients in regimen C were administered on the average 55.7 mg (or 1.1 mg/kg/day) on day 1 and continued to have a slightly higher amount administered on day 4 (117.9 mg/day or 2.4 mg/kg/day) and day 5 (77.3 mg/day or 1.6 mg/kg/day).

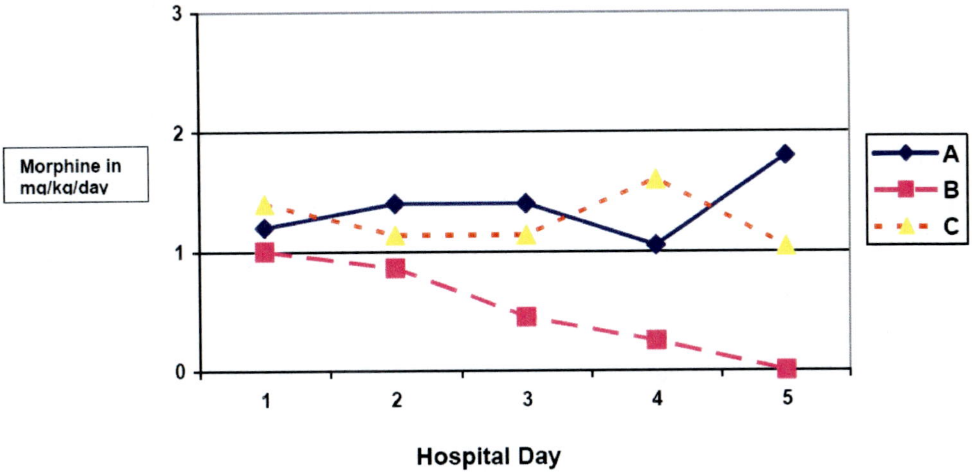

A

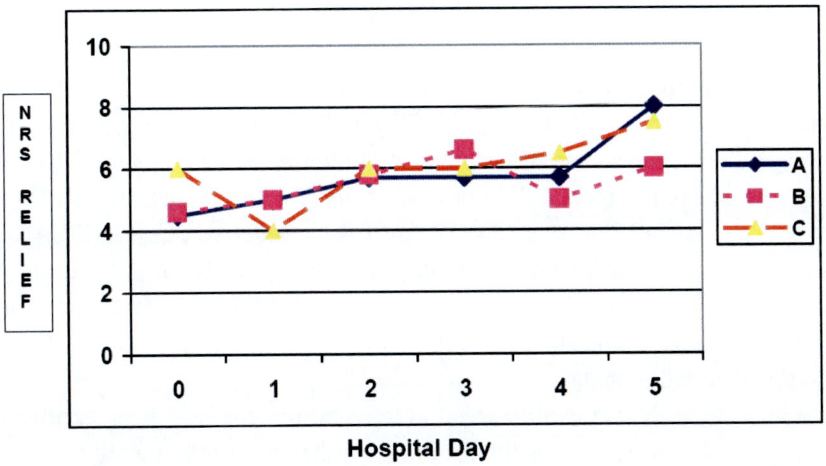

B

Figure 3. Amount of morphine in mg/kg/day (A) and perceived amount of relief [0 to 10 NRS] from medications (B).

Other medications

Ketorolac (administered 15 to 30 mg every 6 hours) was the only other medication that all patients received for pain. A few patients had diphenhydramine for itching, and odansetron (8 mg prn) or promethazine (12 mg prn) for nausea/vomiting.

Pain relief

The amount of pain relief did not change significantly ($p > 0.05$) during hospitalization (figure 3). The mean amount of pain relief (from 0 = no relief to 10 = complete relief) for each day of hospitalization was higher for regimen C (6.0 ± 2.0 to 6.5 ± 2.1), when compared with Regimen A (4.6 ± 2.5 to 5.7 ± 2.1) or B (4.6 ± 2.7 to 6.6 ± 1.9).

Side effects

Few patients were reporting side effects, mostly drowsiness, dizziness, itching, nausea, and vomiting. Two of five patients from regimen A and three of five patients from regimen B reported drowsiness prior to enrollment. Three patients on regimen A and two patients on regimen B also reported itching on day of enrollment. Two patients had nausea from regimen A and one each from regimen B and C had both nausea and vomiting. No one had low blood pressure, heart rate, or respiratory rate. One patient in regimen B had difficulty stooling, reported prior to enrollment.

Discussion

This preliminary study evaluated the analgesic response to three different morphine regimens delivered by patient controlled analgesia (PCA). The worst pain intensity ratings in regimen B decreased during the course of hospitalization, while the worst pain intensity ratings in the other two regimens (A and C) did not change. This finding suggests that the regimen with higher background infusion rate (B) may provide a better response to PCA morphine. The difference in trends between the worst and least pain intensity ratings were also narrower in regimen B, suggesting that pain peaks and troughs were not occurring in regimen B, as they were most likely occurring in regimen C, with wide differences in highest pain and lowest pain ratings reported each day.

It is interesting to note that the trend in least pain intensity ratings reported by patients in regimen C was lower across hospitalization days than reported by patients in either regimen A or B (see figure 2). The difference in trends between the worst and least pain intensity ratings across the hospital days was widest in regimen C. This finding suggests that the higher intermittent doses were providing better relief than the amount that were delivered in either regimen A or B; however the every 3 hour interval was most likely not adequate to sustain the low intensity ratings, and may explain the high pain intensity ratings.

Patients in regimen A were reporting the highest worst and least pain intensity ratings and both remained consistently high throughout hospitalization. This finding is similar to previous reports (9,10), which also reported regimens similar to regimen A and worst and least pain intensity ratings that remained high to moderate throughout hospitalization. This implies that the routinely prescribed PCA regimen with lower background infusion and high intermittent push doses (similar to the doses prescribed in regimen A for this study) was not providing optimal pain control.

The chest, abdomen, and extremities were the most frequently marked areas for pain in all regimens, which are similar to the pain location marked by patients in previous reports (9,10). The number of areas marked decreased for patients in regimens A and B. It is important to note that pain intensity ratings remained at high to moderate levels throughout hospitalization (figure 1A), but the number of body areas marked with pain decreased (figure 1B) for regimen A and B. This finding emphasizes the importance of assessing not only pain intensity dimension as routinely done in practice, but also assessing the location and spatial distribution of pain throughout hospitalization (8), which could be more informative in evaluating response to treatments. This data suggest that regimens A and B were providing better analgesia when compared to regimen C (figure 1B) when the dimension of pain location is used as the outcome criteria.

The most frequently used words selected to describe the quality of pain were predominantly sensory, and less frequently affective, evaluative, or temporal. Patients did not select words that suggest pain with neuropathic component (e.g. shooting, burning, or shock-like). This finding is similar to previous reports of patients with sickle cell disease (8,21).

The amount of morphine prescribed was standardized for all three regimens, which was selected so that the hourly maximum setting is midpoint of the therapeutic dose range (13). We were anticipating that patients in regimen B would consume more morphine since the background infusion rate was higher. However, patients in regimen B showed a consistent decrease in their daily morphine consumption throughout hospitalization (figure 3A). Although not statistically significant, possibly due to small sample size, the length of stay for regimen B is shorter (table 1). This finding is suggesting that a higher background infusion rate (regimen B) than would routinely be prescribed (regimen A) within the first 24 hours of admission for acute painful episode may provide improved response and shorter recovery from the painful episode in patients with sickle cell disease.

An important finding in this study is that on the average, patients in the ED received 0.08 to 0.10 mg/kg/dose, which were lower or within the lower end of the recommended therapeutic dose range of 0.1 to 0.2 mg/kg/dose (13). This finding is similar to previous studies which reported that in children and adolescents with sickle cell disease, the prescribed morphine doses were frequently prescribed and administered in the lower end of the therapeutic dose range (9,10). It would be interesting to determine in future studies whether standardizing the ED protocol to increase the amount prescribed to at least the midpoint of the therapeutic dose range would lead to improved analgesia in the ED and thereby minimize the number of admissions related to acute painful episodes (4,22,23).

The patients in regimen C were reporting a higher relief than patients in regimens A and B. It is possible that the higher intermittent doses administered by the nurse around the clock were providing good relief. These pain relief data are consistent with their reports of least pain intensity ratings.

We did not examine the regimen with high background infusion rate and high intermittent push dose that would be within the therapeutic dose range, a regimen that may be optimal. Future studies need to examine this regimen using larger sample size. There were no differences in side effects reported by patients. The side effects (mostly drowsiness, dizziness, itching, nausea, and vomiting) were present prior to initiation of the doses prescribed in the regimens.

A major limitation in this study is the small sample size. We recommend larger samples in future studies. We screened and recruited patients from the hematology program serving a large population of patients with sickle cell disease. During the two year screening and recruitment period, we were only able to enroll 15 patients (including two early withdrawal patients). We recommend that in future studies, screening and recruitment be done in several sites as the pool of patients with sickle cell disease requiring patient controlled analgesia is relatively low compared to the overall number of all patients with sickle cell disease in a hospital setting.

Several studies including the current study, have documented that the most routinely prescribed regimen (similar to the doses prescribed in Regimen A with high intermittent push with low background infusion rates) was not optimal in providing analgesia. Our current study also showed that patients prescribed a nurse administered around the clock q 3 hour regimen (as prescribed in regimen C) were most likely experiencing pain peaks and troughs, and therefore such regimens should be avoided. We recommend future studies to examine a high background infusion rate with low intermittent push dose (as was prescribed for regimen B) and alternative morphine regimens such as high background infusion with high intermittent push dose, while keeping within the recommended dose range (13). Previous reports have documented that patients with sickle cell disease required higher dosing schedules due to the more intense pain (24), prolonged hospitalizations (10), and altered pharmacokinetics (25). And finally, future studies are warranted that examine alternative PCA opioids such as hydromorphone (26), fentanyl (27), tramadol (28) or a combination of morphine and an adjuvant medication such as ketamine (29) in patients with sickle cell disease who experience severe pain that may be refractory to morphine PCA.

Acknowledgments

Funding from this study was provided by a Mentored Patient-Oriented Research Career Development Award (#5K23NR009192) from the National Institute of Nursing Research at the National Institute of Health.

References

[1] Platt OS, Brambilla DJ, Rosse WF, Milner PF, Castro O, Steinberg MH et al. Mortality in sickle cell disease. Life expectancy and risk factors for early death. N Engl J Med 1994;330(23):1639-44.

[2] Platt OS, Thorington BD, Brambilla DJ, Milner PF, Rosse WF, Vichinsky E et al. Pain in sickle cell disease. Rates and risk factors. N Engl J Med 1991;325(1):11-16.

[3] Yang Y, Sha A, Watson M, Mankad V. Comparison of costs to the health sector of comprehensive and episodic health care for sickle cell disease patients. Public Health Reports 1997;110:80-6.

[4] Blank FSJ, Li, H, Henneman, PL, Smithline, HA, Santoro, JS, Provost, D, Maynard, AM. A descriptive study of heavy emergency department users at an academic emergency department reveals heavy ED users have better access to care than average users. J Emerg Nurs 2005;31(2):139-44.

[5] Beyer J, Simmons L, Woods GM, Woods PM. A chronology of pain/comfort in children with sickle cell disease. Arch Pediatr Adolesc Med 1999;153(9):913-20.

[6] Ballas S. The acute painful episode. In: Sickle cell pain. Seattle: IASP Press 1998;11:201-37.

[7] Conner-Warren RL. Pain intensity and home pain management of children with sickle cell disease. Issues Compr Pediatr Nurs 1996;19(3):183-95.

[8] Jacob E, Miaskowski C, Savedra M, Beyer JE, Treadwell M, Styles L. Changes in intensity, location, and quality of vaso-occlusive pain. Pain 2003;102(1-2):187-93.

[9] Jacob E, Miaskowski C, Savedra M, Beyer JE, Treadwell M, Styles L. Management of vaso-occlusive pain in hospitalized children with sickle cell disease. J Pediatr Hematology/Oncology 2003;25(4):307-11.

[10] Jacob E, Mueller B. Pain and symptom experience in hospitalized children with sickle cell disease who had prolonged hospitalizations. Pain Med 01 Feb 2007 [EPub ahead of print]

[11] Sutters KA, Miaskowski C, Holdridge-Zeuner D, Waite S, Paul SM, Savedra MC, Lanier B. A randomized clinical trial of the effectiveness of a scheduled oral analgesic dosing regimen for the management of postoperative pain in children following tonsillectomy. Pain 20041;110(1-2):49-55.

[12] Sutters KA, Miaskowski C, Holdridge-Zeuner D, Waite S, Paul SM, Savedra MC, Lanier B. Time-contingent dosing of an opioid analgesic after tonsillectomy does not increase moderate-to-severe side effects in children. Pain Manag Nurs 2005;6(2):49-57.

[13] Taketomo CK, Hodding JH, Kraus DM. Pediatric dosage handbook. Hudson, Ohio: Lexi-comp, 2007.

[14] Brunton L, Lazo J, Lazo, JS. Goodman and Gilman's the Pharmacological basis of therapeutics, 11th ed. New York: McGraw-Hill, 2005:569-20.

[15] Benjamin LJ, Dampier CD, Jacox AK, Odesina V, Phoenix D, Shapiro B et al. Guideline for the management of acute and chronic pain in sickle cell disease. Glenview, Ill: Am Pain Society, 1999:42.

[16] Burns N, Groves S. The practice of nursing research. Philadelphia, PA: WB Saunders, 2003:292.

[17] Savedra M, Tesler M, Holzemer WL, Wilkie DJ, Ward JA. Testing a tool to assess postoperative pediatric and adolescent pain. In: Tyler DC, Krane EJ, eds. Advances in pain research and therapy: Pediatric pain. New York: Raven Press, 1990.

[18] Savedra MC, Holzemer WL, Tesler MD, Wilkie DJ. Assessment of postoperation pain in children and adolescents using the adolescent pediatric pain tool. Nurs Res 1993;42(1):5-9.

[19] Savedra MC, Tesler MD, Holzemer WL, Wilkie DJ, Ward JA. Pain location: Validity and reliability of body outline markings by hospitalized children and adolescents. Res Nurs Health 1989;12: 307-14.

[20] Wilkie DJ, Holzemer WL, Tesler MD, Ward JA, Paul SM, Savedra MC. Measuring pain quality: Validity and reliability of children's and adolescents' pain language. Pain 1990;41:151-9.

[21] Franck LS, Treadwell M, Jacob E, Vichinsky E. Assessment of sickle cell pain in children and young adults using the adolescent pediatric pain tool. J Pain Sympt Manage 2002;23:114-20.

[22] Givens M, Rutherford C, Joshi G, Delaney K. Impact of an emergency department pain management protocol on the pattern of visits by patients with sickle cell disease. J Emerg Med 2006;32(3):239-43.

[23] Melzer-Lange MD, Walsh-Kelly CM, Lean G, Hillery CA, Scott JP. Patient-controlled analgesia for sickle cell pain crisis in a pediatric emergency department. Pediatr Emerg Care 2004;20(1):2-4.

[24] Crawford MC, Galton S, Naser B. Postoperative morphine consumption in children with sickle cell disease. Pediatric Anesthesia 2006;16:152-7.

[25] Dampier CD, Setty BN, Logan J, Ioli JG, Dean R. Intravenous morphine pharmacokinetics in pediatric patients with sickle cell disease. J Pediatr 1995;126(3):461-7.

[26] Perlman KM, Myers-Phariss S, Rhodes JC. A shift from meperidine to hydromorphone improves pain control and decreases admissions for patients in sickle cell crisis. 2004;30(5):439-46.

[27] Ruggiero A, Barone G, Liotti L, Chiaretti A, Lazzareschi I, Riccardi R. Safety and efficacy of fentanyl administered by patient controlled analgesia in children with cancer pain. Supportive Care Cancer 2007;15:569-73.

[28] Ozalevli M, Unlugenc H, Tuncer U, Gunes Y, Ozcengiz D. Comparison of morphine and tramadol by patient controlled analgesia for postoperative analgesia after tonsillectomy in children. Pediatric Anesthesia 2005;15:979-84.

[29] Subramaniam K, Subramaniam B, Stenbrook RA. Ketamine as adjuvant analgesic to opioids: A quantitative and qualitative systematic review. Anesthesia Analgesia 2004;99:482-95.

IV. Coping with pain in healthy children

In: Children and Pain
Editors: P. Schofield and J. Merrick

ISBN 978-1-60876-020-6

Chapter 6

Healthy children's experimental pain responses

Subhadra Evans**, PhD, Qian Lu, MD, PhD, Jennie CI Tsao, PhD and Lonnie K Zeltzer, MD
Pediatric Pain Program, Department of Pediatrics,
David Geffen School of Medicine,
University of California Los Angeles,
Los Angeles, California, United States

Abstract

This chapter examine the relationship between race, laboratory-based coping strategies and anticipatory anxiety and pain intensity for cold, thermal (heat) and pressure experimental pain tasks. Participants were 123 healthy children and adolescents, including 33 African Americans (51% female; mean age =13.9 years) and 90 Caucasians (50% female; mean age = 12.6 years). Coping in response to the cold task was assessed with the Lab Coping Style interview; based on their interview responses, participants were categorized as 'attenders' (i.e., those who focused on the task) vs. 'distractors' (i.e., those who distracted themselves during the task). Analysis of covariance (ANCOVA) revealed significant interactions between race (African-American vs. Caucasian) and lab-based coping style after controlling for sex, age and socioeconomic status. African-American children classified as attenders reported less anticipatory anxiety for the cold task and lower pain intensity for the cold, heat and pressure tasks compared to those categorized as distractors. For these pain outcomes, Caucasian children classified as distractors reported less anticipatory anxiety and lower pain intensity relative to those categorized as attenders. The findings point to the moderating effect of coping in the relationship between race and experimental pain sensitivity.

---

* Correspondence: Subhadra Evans, PhD, Pediatric Pain Program, Department of Pediatrics, David Geffen School of Medicine at UCLA, 10940 Wilshire Blvd., Suite 810, Los Angeles, California 90024. Tel: 310-794 2936; Fax: 310 794 2954; E-mail: suevans@mednet.ucla.edu.

Introduction

Racial and ethnic differences in the experience of pain have long been noted. Numerous investigators have reported racial/ethnic disparities in adult studies of clinical pain (1-4) and laboratory pain (5-7). For the most part, these findings show that, compared to Caucasians, African Americans report higher levels of pain, including pain unpleasantness, emotional reactions to pain, higher pain intensity and lower pain threshold. In addition, it appears that African Americans evidence distinct methods of pain coping, which together with increased levels of pain-related anxiety and depression, may contribute towards marked pain sensitivity (1). However, limited research has examined the influence of race/ethnicity on children's pain sensitivity.

The present chapter attempts to address the current gap in our knowledge of racial differences in pain and coping among children—a topic of clear import, given that an individual's ideas about race/ethnicity, pain and coping are all formed early in life (8, 9). Not to preclude the possible role of biology in racial/ethnic differences in pain (7), but racial/ethnic identity reflects to a large degree sociocultural and family processes, making the relationships among race/ethnicity, pain and coping especially noteworthy early in the developmental trajectory.

Two strands of adult research show that coping is intricately linked to an individual's experience of pain. The first documents an association between general coping style and pain, such that the tendency to use passive or external coping strategies is associated with higher pain sensitivity (10, 11), and moreover, that African Americans tend to report different coping preferences to Caucasians (1,12,13). The second strand has examined coping in response to a particular pain episode, revealing that for some populations and pain conditions, attending to pain is often less effective than distracting oneself from pain (14). Similar to the adult literature, children who use distraction to cope with acute laboratory pain are more likely to report increased pain tolerance (15), particularly when instruction to use distraction is concordant with the child's natural coping methods (16). As yet it is unclear whether there are racial/ethnic differences in the tendency to divert or avert attention in the laboratory pain setting, and the use of coping strategies is untested in children of different racial/ethnic backgrounds.

We conducted the present study to investigate African American and Caucasian children's laboratory-specific coping and pain in response to experimental pain tasks. The focus on laboratory specific coping is consistent with the idea that coping is likely to be situation and pain- specific (17). Racial/ethnic-coping relationships in the context of experimental pain are likely to vary depending on whether general coping versus situation-specific coping is assessed (5). Given that experimental pain situations are relatively unique in the child's pain experience, it was deemed important to assess their lab-specific pain coping. To our knowledge, this study is the first to examine racial/ethnic differences in coping and laboratory pain in a sample of children. Three laboratory pain modalities were used: pressure, thermal heat, and cold pain.

Given the paucity of previous research, no directional hypotheses were advanced. However, based on the adult literature, it was anticipated that distinct patterns for laboratory-based coping and pain responses would emerge for African American and Caucasian children.

Our sample

The current sample was drawn from a larger sample of 240 children who participated in a study on the effects of gender and puberty on laboratory pain responses described previously (18). The initial sample included five different racial/ethnic categories, including 'Hispanic' (n = 57), 'Asian/Pacific Islander' (n = 24) and 'Other (n = 30).' Due to the focus on African American and Caucasian participants in the previous adult literature, only African American and Caucasian participants were included in this analysis. Thus, the present study included 98 Caucasians and 34 African Americans. Nine participants who reported no coping strategy on the coping style interview (described below) were removed. One-way ANOVAs and chi square statistics revealed no significant differences in age, sex or race between the 9 participants who reported no coping strategy and the participants included in the current study. The final sample consisted of 123 healthy children (50% male): 90 Caucasians (73%) and 33 African Americans (27%). Mean age was 12.9 years (SD, 2.97 years) and mean grade in school was 7th grade. Participant demographics for each racial group are presented in Table 1.

Participants were recruited from a major urban area through posted advertisements, mass mailing and classroom presentations. Recruitment was targeted at various racial/ethnic groups across sites of varied socioeconomic status. Telephone screening reduced an initial 489 interested individuals to 244 eligible participants, with four failing to complete the study due to time and constraints (n = 3) and discomfort with being attached to the electrodes (n = 1). The University of California, Los Angeles (UCLA) Institutional Review board (IRB), as well as the IRBs for recruitment sites approved all recruitment and study procedures.

Table 1. Demographic and coping information by race

	African Americans		Caucasians	
Age	13.89 (3.25)		12.60 (2.80)*	
Sex	Males: 16 (49%) Females: 17 (51%) n		Males: 45 (50%) Females: 45 (50%) n	
Parent Education Level	Partial High School	1	Partial High School	0
	High School Graduate	12	High School Graduate	8
	Partial college	9	Partial college	12
	Bachelor's degree	5	Bachelor's degree	38
	Graduate degree	1	Graduate degree	31*
Parent Occupation	51 (13.01)		74 (13.17)*	
Lab Coping Style	Attender: 24 (73%) Distractor: 9 (27%)		Attender: 54 (57%) Distractor: 36 (33%)	

Unless otherwise specified African American n = 33, Caucasian n = 90.
* $p < .05$.

The pain tasks selected have been previously performed with children without adverse effects. IRB approved consent and assent forms were completed by parents and children. Participants received a $30 video store voucher and a t-shirt for their participation.

Procedure

Each participant visited the testing site once. Upon visiting the laboratory, participants completed demographic and psychosocial questionnaires with an experimenter in a room adjacent to the laboratory. Two experimenters conducted the sessions; experimenters included five females and two males. A male experimenter conducted the study with 4 participants, with female experimenters conducting the sessions on the other occasions. There were no differences between racial groups in the presence of male vs. female experimenters (X2 = .01, p>.05).

After completing the questionnaires, participants were escorted to the laboratory where they completed three pain tasks, namely cold pressor, thermal heat and cutaneous pressure tasks (described below). Prior to the administration of the pain tasks, participants were instructed on the use of a vertical sliding visual analog scale (VAS) for rating pain intensity and anticipatory anxiety (described below). More detailed descriptions of the procedure, including randomization and ordering of tasks have been reported previously(18, 19). Immediately, after the cold pressor task (CPT), the pain coping strategy interview, which assessed what subjects did or thought about to keep their hand immersed longer and which strategy was employed the most was administered to determine the primary laboratory-based coping style.

Laboratory pain tasks

Cold pressor task

Participants underwent a single trial of 10 ?C water using a commercial ice chest measuring 38 cm wide, 71 cm long and 35 cm deep. A plastic mesh screen separated crushed ice from a plastic large-hole mesh armrest in the cold water. Water was circulated through the ice by a pump to prevent local warming about the hand. Participants were instructed to keep the dominant hand in cold water to a depth of 2" above the wrist for as long as they could. The task had an uninformed ceiling of 3 minutes, and participants were asked to keep their hand in for as long as they could, but were informed they may be told to take their hand out sooner.

Pressure task

The Ugo Basile Analgesy-Meter 37215 (Ugo Basile Biological Research Apparatus, Comerio, Italy) was used to administer focal pressure through a lucite point approximately 1.5 mm in diameter to the second dorsal phalanx of the middle finger and index finger of each hand. Four trials, two at each of two levels of pressure (322.5 g and 465 g), were run with an uninformed ceiling of 3 minutes. Participants were instructed that they would experience pressure and to leave their finger in place for as long as possible, and they were free to remove the weight at any time.

Thermal heat task

The Ugo Basile 7360 Unit (Ugo Basile Biological Research Apparatus, Comerio, Italy) was used to administer four trials of two infrared stimulus intensities (15, 20) of radiant heat 2 inches proximal to the wrist and 3 inches distal to the elbow on both volar forearms with an uninformed ceiling of 20 seconds. Participants were informed that the task would involve heat and some discomfort, shown where to place their forearm and told they could move their arm away at any time.

Pain outcome measures

For each task, anticipatory anxiety and pain intensity were assessed. Participants were asked to rate pain intensity and anticipatory anxiety using a visual analog scale (VAS). The VAS was rated using a vertical slider, which was anchored with 0 at one end, and 10 at the other. The scale also included corresponding color cues, from white to dark red. The VAS is brief, easily understood and possesses excellent psychometric properties(20).

Anticipatory anxiety was obtained through participants' visual analogue scale (VAS) ratings in response to the instruction 'how nervous, afraid, or worried' they were about the upcoming task. Pain intensity was assessed immediately after each trial by asking participants to use the VAS to rate the amount of pain they experienced during the task. Specifically, participants were asked 'at its worst, how much pain did you feel?'

Psychological measures

Pain coping

Lab Coping Style Interview assessed the specific coping style children favored in response to cold pain. The experimenter asked the following: 'Some kids think or do certain things while their hand is in the water; What did you do or think about to make it easier to keep your hand in the water longer?' Children's responses were tape-recorded and then transcribed verbatim. Participants' responses were categorized by two independent raters as either "attenders" or "distractors" based on the primary coping strategy used. This procedure was consistent with the methodology and definitions used previously to distinguish attenders from distractors(15, 16). Inter-rater reliability for assignment to groups was obtained for two raters (Kappa = .96).

Attenders were classified as those who focused their attention toward the task, such as through paying attention to sensory information, focusing on the task, or focusing on any attempts to cope with discomfort. Distractors were classified as those who diverted attention away from the sensations or emotional reactions related to the task, including visual, mental and physical distraction, imagery and relaxation/ breathing.

Demographic variables

A locally developed demographic information questionnaire was given to care-givers who brought their child to the laboratory to participate in the study. The questionnaire assessed demographic information about the child, including age, sex, race/ethnicity, and demographic information about the child's mother and father, including education attained, occupation and household income. A composite variable was computed for mother and father education, as well as a combined mother/father occupation score using the occupation code from Hollingshead Index of Social Status(21). Occupation was classified into one of nine categories (0-90), with increasingly higher numeric scores denoting increasingly higher occupational status. Codes can be used categorically to determine social class or continuously, with higher scores representing higher status employment. The education variable is representative of parents' education level, with higher scores indicating greater education attainment. The average education score and average occupation score were used as proxy variables for socioeconomic status (SES). Due to the large number of missing data for household income (missing n = 101), this variable was not used in analyses.

Statistical analysis

Independent samples t-tests for continuous data and chi-square tests for categorical data were used to examine mean differences between African Americans and Caucasians on demographic variables. Confirmatory analyses using 2 (race: African American vs. Caucasian) X 2 (coping style: attender vs. distractor) ANCOVAs on laboratory pan outcomes were conducted, controlling for demographic covariates that differed between the racial groups. Separate ANCOVAs were conducted for each of the pain outcomes (anticipatory anxiety; pain intensity) for each pain task (cold, pressure and heat). The ANCOVAs tested the main effects of race and of coping style as well as the interaction between race and coping style on the pain outcomes. Significant interaction effects were examined using post hoc Sidak tests on the marginal means to delineate the simple effects. General linear modeling was also used to plot significant interactions and examine simple effects.

Pain intensity ratings for the thermal and pressure tasks were highly correlated across the four trials within each task (r's = .73 - .83, $p < .001$). Similarly, anticipatory anxiety ratings for the thermal and pressure tasks were highly correlated across the four trials within each task (r's = .59 - .71, $p < .001$). Pain intensity ratings and anticipatory anxiety ratings for the thermal and pressure tasks were therefore averaged across the four trials within each task yielding a single mean value for pressure intensity, heat intensity, pressure anticipatory anxiety, and heat anticipatory anxiety.

Results

Racial differences in demographics and coping

Table 1 shows descriptive statistics for each racial group. There were a number of significant differences on the demographic variables between African Americans and Caucasians. African American children were significantly older than Caucasians ($t = 2.16$, $p = .03$); parents of African American children were less likely to attain a higher level of formal education (X2 = 56.63, $p = .00$) and have higher occupation status ($t = 6.65$, $p = .00$) compared to parents of Caucasian children. There were no differences in lab coping style categories by race. Although relative percentages indicated that a higher proportion of African Americans were categorized as attenders compared to Caucasians, this difference was not significant.

Relationships between coping and race

Given the demographic differences between the groups, SES, age and sex were entered as covariates in the ANCOVAs on the pain outcomes. Results of the ANCOVAs including F ratios and p values are reported in Table 3. Marginal means with results from post-hoc Sidak tests for each pain outcome are presented in table 3. The raw means for the pain outcomes by race are presented in table 2. The ANCOVAs indicated a significant main effect for coping on cold intensity only, with distracters reporting higher cold intensity compared to attenders. There were no other significant main effects. Significant race by coping interactions were found for cold anticipatory anxiety, cold intensity, heat intensity and pressure intensity (see table 3). All the interactions displayed the same pattern; attending was associated with lower levels of pain for African Americans compared to distracting, while distracting was associated with lower levels of pain for Caucasians relative to attending.

Table 2. Raw mean (*SD*) scores for pain outcomes by race and coping style

Pain Outcome		African Americans	Caucasians
Cold Anticipatory Anxiety (VAS)	Attender:	1.44 (2.86)	2.33 (2.46)
	Distractor:	4.27 (3.26)	1.99 (1.89)
Cold Intensity (VAS)	Attender:	1.83 (2.30)	4.01 (3.04)
	Distractor:	6.52 (3.77)	2.94 (2.44)
Heat Anticipatory Anxiety (VAS)	Attender:	2.58 (2.19)	4.64 (2.90)
	Distractor:	4.61 (2.78)	3.80 (2.70)
Heat Intensity (VAS)	Attender:	2.74 (1.84)	5.54 (2.68)
	Distractor:	5.93 (2.60)	5.04 (2.59)
Pressure Anticipatory Anxiety (VAS)	Attender:	2.34 (2.29)	3.61 (2.33)
	Distractor:	4.44 (3.03)	2.89 (2.28)
Pressure Intensity (VAS)	Attender:	3.74 (2.50)	5.59 (2.59)
	Distractor:	6.33 (2.33)	4.45 (2.43)

Table 3. Results of the ANCOVAs on the marginal means for pain outcomes controlling for sex, age and SES

Dependent Variables	Independent Variables	Marginal mean (SE)		*F (DF)*	*P*
Cold Anticipatory Anxiety	Race	Caucasian	2.13 (.29)	.87 (1)	.35
		African Am	2.96 (.81)		
	Coping	Attender	1.92 (.39)	2.64 (1)	.11
		Distractor	3.17 (.69)		
	Race X Coping	Caucasian Attender	2.30 (.38)	4.39 (1)	.04*
		Caucasian Distractor	1.96 (.44)		
		African Am Attender	1.56 (.76)		
		African Am Distractor	4.37 (1.31)		
Cold Intensity	Race	Caucasian	3.49 (.32)	.26 (1)	.43
		African Am	4.02 (.90)		
	Coping	Attender	2.90 (.44)	4.07 (1)	.04*
		Distractor	4.61 (.77)		
	Race X Coping	Caucasian Attender	4.10 (.43)	11.92 (1)	.00**
		Caucasian Distractor	2.88 (.49)		
		African Am Attender	1.70 (.84)		
		African Am Distractor	6.34 (1.5)		
Heat Anticipatory Anxiety	Race	Caucasian	4.21 (.33)	.30	.59
		African Am	3.66 (.91)		
	Coping	Attender	3.63 (.45)	.51	.48
		Distractor	4.24 (.78)		
	Race X Coping	Caucasian Attender	4.62 (.43)	2.83	.09
		Caucasian Distractor	3.81 (.49)		
		African Am Attender	2.64 (.85)		
		African Am Distractor	4.67 (1.48)		
Heat Intensity	Race	Caucasian	5.24 (.30)	.43	.51
		African Am	4.62 (.85)		
	Coping	Attender	4.22 (.41)	3.12	.08
		Distractor	5.63 (.72)		
	Race X Coping	Caucasian Attender	5.44 (.40)	5.39	.02*
		Caucasian Distractor	5.03 (.46)		
		African Am Attender	3.00 (.79)		
		African Am Distractor	6.24 (1.37)		
Pressure Anticipatory Anxiety	Race	Caucasian	3.30 (.28)	.04	.84
		African Am	3.13 (.77)		
	Coping	Attender	2.91 (.38)	.70	.40
		Distractor	3.52 (.66)		
	Race X Coping	Caucasian Attender	3.65 (.37)	3.39	.07
		Caucasian Distractor	2.95 (.42)		
		African Am Attender	2.17 (.72)		
		African Am Distractor	4.09 (1.25)		
Pressure Intensity	Race	Caucasian	5.10 (.30)	.41	.52
		African Am	4.51 (.84)		
	Coping	Attender	4.57 (.41)	.36	.55
		Distractor	5.04 (.71)		
	Race X Coping	Caucasian Attender	5.76 (.40)	5.28	.02*
		Caucasian Distractor	4.45 (.45)		
		African Am Attender	3.39 (.78)		
		African Am Distractor	5.65 (1.35)		

(*p< .05).

Significant interactions between ethnicity and coping

General linear modeling was used to plot the significant race by coping interactions, controlling for sex, age and SES. Figures 1-4 show the interactions.

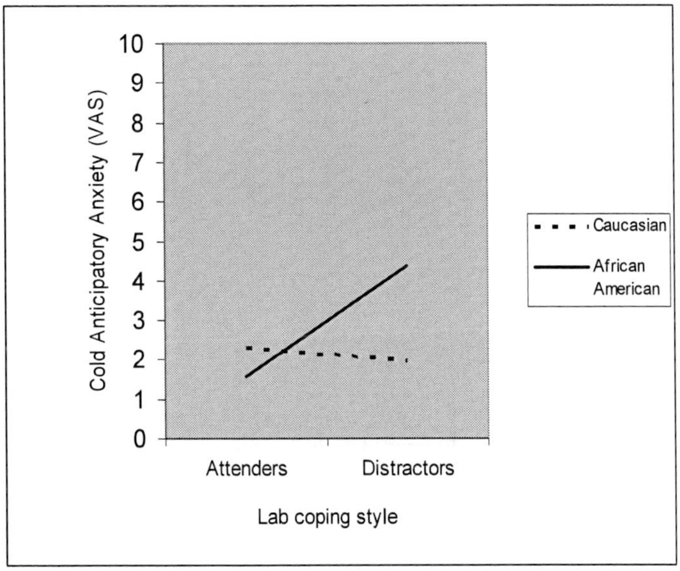

Figure 1. Significant interaction between race and lab coping for cold anticipatory anxiety controlling for sex, age and SES.

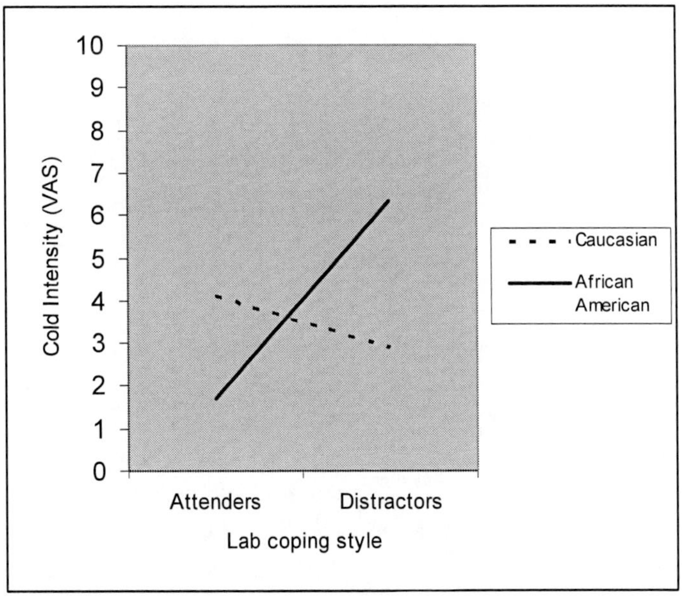

Figure 2. Significant interaction between race and lab coping for cold intensity controlling for sex, age and SES.

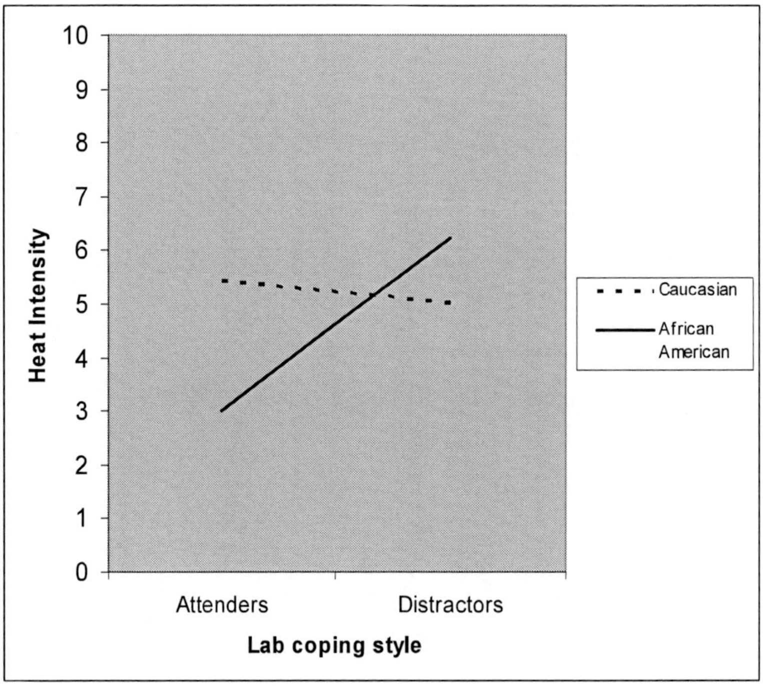

Figure 3. Significant interaction between race and lab coping for heat intensity controlling for sex, age and SES.

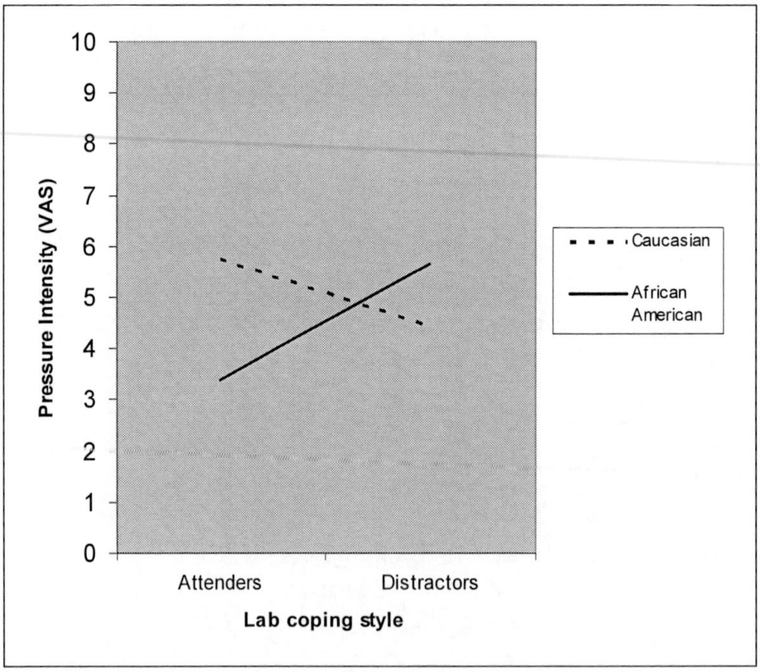

Figure 4. Significant interaction between race and lab coping for pressure intensity controlling for sex, age and SES.

The relationship between race and coping was consistent across cold anticipatory anxiety, cold intensity, heat intensity and pressure intensity. For African Americans, attending to the pain situation was associated with lower pain sensitivity compared to distraction. In contrast, Caucasians who attended to pain reported increased pain sensitivity, relative to distraction. Analysis of simple effects using general linear modeling revealed that, relative to Caucasian attenders, African Americans attenders reported significantly lower cold intensity ($F(1,87)= 5.71$, $p <.05$), pressure intensity ($F(1,87)= 6.59$, $p <.05$), and heat intensity ($F(1,87)= 6.79$, $p <.05$). In addition, African American distractors reported significantly higher cold intensity than Caucasian distractors ($F(1,87)= 5.06$, $p <.05$).

Discussion

This study demonstrated a relationship between laboratory-based coping, race and experimental pain sensitivity in healthy children. A number of significant interaction effects were demonstrated after controlling for sex as well as age and SES differences between the groups. In African-Americans, a distracting coping style was associated with increased pain responses relative to attending, whereas in Caucasians, a distracting coping style was related to decreased pain responses compared to attending. It appears that lab-based coping style moderates the impact of race on children's experimental cold, heat and pressure pain responses.

Previous findings relating to the efficacy of distraction versus attention for pain management in healthy individuals are mixed. While distraction appears to decrease pain intensity in adults undergoing cold pressor laboratory pain (22) and pressure pain (23), some studies have found attending to sensations is effective in reducing the pain of childbirth (24) and is superior to distraction in coping with cold pressor pain distress (25). The small number of pain coping studies focusing on children and adolescents have also produced mixed findings. Distraction may be superior in reducing cold pain in younger children, while attending and distraction appear to be equally effective for children older than 10 years of age (26). However, other research has found that children are best able to manage cold pressor pain when they are taught coping strategies consistent with their natural tendencies (16). That is, natural distractors exhibited lower pain responses when taught distraction skills but demonstrated increased pain responses when taught to attend, and vice versa for natural attenders. The results of the present study may qualify previous research. The current results indicate that different pain coping styles may be effective for children of different backgrounds. Previous studies may have produced conflicting results by not accounting for individual differences such as race or ethnicity.

Pain-coping moderators that have been considered in previous literature may shed light on the race-coping interactions found here. One such moderator includes length of task, such that distraction may be most effective in reducing laboratory pain early in the procedure with attending effective for longer trials, perhaps due to a temporary 'blocking' effect of pain during distraction, versus an 'interpretation' of the pain during attending that allows for a mitigation of sensations over time (27). It is possible that African American children develop similar 'interpretation' strategies regardless of pain trial length. Distraction further appears to be effective for low pain-fearful individuals, while attending to pain sensations is effective for high pain-fearful individuals, a finding that is consistent for acute laboratory pain (28) and chronic pain (29). It is possible that due to higher stress levels associated with minority status, African-American children may be more fearful of stress and pain situations, leading to the effective use of attending as a pain coping strategy. Although we found no racial differences in anticipatory anxiety, previous studies have used more general measures of health anxiety and pain-related fear rather than anxiety specific to the pain task. Future studies should explore possible mechanisms behind the interaction between race and coping, including racial differences in health-related fear.

Racial differences in general coping styles have been documented in the adult literature, with African Americans tending to use passive coping styles such as catastrophizing, a style that increases the attentional focus on pain (1,12,13) and Caucasians tending to use more active techniques including ignoring pain (12). We found no significant racial differences in coping strategy classifications and no main effects for race, indicating that African American children were no more sensitive to pain than were Caucasian children, and no more likely to use a particular coping strategy. However, when coping and race were considered together, a specific picture emerged for African Americans and Caucasians that was relatively consistent across pain tasks.

Whether such interactions are long-lasting cannot be answered without longitudinal studies following the pain and coping responses of children of different races. Research is also needed to address why and how such differences arise. What is it about being an African American child that leads to increased anxiety and greater pain sensitivity in response to acute pain stimuli when using distraction, and conversely, for Caucasian children attending to the pain experience? As mentioned, future research should examine how life experiences may lead to such relationships. The family may also prove to be an important explanatory force. Parents of different races may model specific coping styles, which could be explored in research examining how parents react to their own and their child's laboratory pain.

It is possible that the race by coping interactions seen here represent an early unfolding of the divergent pain sensitivity found in African American and Caucasian adults. Although there were no main effects for race, our finding that African American children using attending were more likely to experience reduced pain compared to Caucasian children who used attending may provide clues as to why African American adults tend to experience greater laboratory and clinical pain than do Caucasian adults (10).

In childhood, increased attention to pain may elicit greater relief for African Americans, especially during acute pain situations. Over time, attending to pain may prove less effective, with a corresponding increase in pain sensitivity in African Americans. Recently, it has been argued that the benefits of attending to pain may diminish with exposure to pain, such that attending to pain is not effective for those with previous pain experiences (14). Attending may initially be effective for African American children, but prove less so with repeated exposure to pain. Given evidence suggesting the stability of preferred coping styles developed in childhood (15), it may be difficult to adopt other coping strategies if attending to pain has previously proven rewarding.

It is possible that the interactions found here would not extend to other measures of pain sensitivity. Both lab coping and pain intensity reports are based on recall directly after the pain tasks and immediate memory of the pain could potentially influence the reports. Further, choosing to either attend to sensations or distract oneself is likely to have an impact on attentional capacity to perceive pain, and hence, the degree of intensity an individual reports. Lab coping style also showed an interaction with race in predicting anticipatory anxiety for cold pressor pain. Anticipatory anxiety is a proximal measure of the perceived aversiveness of the pain task, and is involved in the pain experience. Neuroimaging studies have shown similar brain activity during the anticipatory and processing stages of pain stimuli (30). Pain processing often involves expectations based on previous experiences of pain, and anticipatory anxiety is one way of assessing this.

A limitation of the study is the failure to include a wider range of pain variables, including threshold. The present findings demonstrate that certain aspects of pain are more likely to show a relationship to race and coping, and it is possible that pain threshold would have also demonstrated a relationship, since attention is involved in both pain coping and first reported pain. A number of other limitations temper the study's conclusions. Primarily, the lab specific pain coping measure was only assessed in response to the cold pain task and it is possible that different strategies would have emerged for the pressure and heat tasks. Another limitation is that coping style was categorized in a dichotomous fashion. It may be that the construct of coping style is best represented by a continuum.

In addition, coping was categorized based on the primary coping style whereas, coping choices may be more complex involving overlap between attending and distracting. With regards to participants, equal numbers in both racial groups and the inclusion of a wider range of races would have provided richer findings. Although the assessment of SES was a strength of the study, it is possible that other proxy measures of SES would have been more accurate. Generally, a child's SES can only be inferred through parental variables. Family income may have provided a more global measure of SES than parental education level and occupation status.

Despite the limitations, this study addresses a significant gap in the literature. While there has been limited attention to the role of psychosocial variables in the ethnicity-pain relationship (5), the intersection of pain, ethnicity and psychosocial variables has gone entirely unexamined in children and adolescents. It appears that children's pain coping is not 'one size fits all.' It is important for researchers and clinicians to consider potential moderators in the experience of pain. Variables such as race, ethnicity, coping and their interactions may contribute to varied pain responses in children and adults. The present study represents a starting point to understanding how coping strategies may serve different children in their experience of pain.

Acknowledgments

This study was supported by 2R01DE012754 (PI: Lonnie K. Zeltzer) awarded by the National Institute of Dental and Craniofacial Research

References

[1] Cano A, Mayo A, Ventimiglia M. Coping, pain severity, interference, and disability: the potential mediating and moderating roles of race and education. J Pain 2006;7(7):459-68.
[2] Hastie BA, Riley JL, Fillingim RB. Ethnic differences and responses to pain in healthy young adults. Pain Med 2005;6(1):61-71.
[3] Green CR, Baker TA, Sato Y, Washington TL, Smith EM. Race and chronic pain: A comparative study of young black and white Americans presenting for management. J Pain 2003;4(4):176-83.
[4] Green CR, Baker TA, Smith EM, Sato Y. The effect of race in older adults presenting for chronic pain management: a comparative study of black and white Americans. J Pain 2003;4(2):82-90.
[5] Campbell CM, Edwards RR, Fillingim RB. Ethnic differences in responses to multiple experimental pain stimuli. Pain 2005;113(1-2):20-6.
[6] Kim H, Neubert JK, San Miguel A, Xu K, Krishnaraju RK, Iadarola MJ et al. Genetic influence on variability in human acute experimental pain sensitivity associated with gender, ethnicity and psychological temperament. Pain 2004;109(3):488-96.
[7] Mechlin MB, Maixner W, Light KC, Fisher JM, Girdler SS. African Americans show alterations in endogenous pain regulatory mechanisms and reduced pain tolerance to experimental pain procedures. Psychosom Med 2005;67(6):948-56.
[8] Rahim-Williams FB, Riley JL, 3rd, Herrera D, Campbell CM, Hastie BA, Fillingim RB. Ethnic identity predicts experimental pain sensitivity in African Americans and Hispanics. Pain 2007;129(1-2):177-84.
[9] Zimmer-Gembeck MJ, Locke EM. The socialization of adolescent coping behaviours: relationships with families and teachers. J Adolesc 2007;30(1):1-16.
[10] Edwards RR, Moric M, Husfeldt B, Buvanendran A, Ivankovich O. Ethnic similarities and differences in the chronic pain experience: a comparison of african american, Hispanic, and white patients. Pain Med 2005;6(1):88-98.
[11] Lame IE, Peters ML, Vlaeyen JW, Kleef M, Patijn J. Quality of life in chronic pain is more associated with beliefs about pain, than with pain intensity. Eur J Pain 2005;9(1):15-24.
[12] Jordan MS, Lumley MA, Leisen JC. The relationships of cognitive coping and pain control beliefs to pain and adjustment among African-American and Caucasian women with rheumatoid arthritis. Arthritis Care Res 1998;11(2):80-8.
[13] Tan G, Jensen MP, Thornby J, Anderson KO. Ethnicity, control appraisal, coping, and adjustment to chronic pain among black and white Americans. Pain Med 2005;6(1):18-28.
[14] Nouwen A, Cloutier C, Kappas A, Warbrick T, Sheffield D. Effects of focusing and distraction on cold pressor-induced pain in chronic back pain patients and control subjects. J Pain 2006;7(1):62-71.
[15] Tsao JC, Fanurik D, Zeltzer LK. Long-term effects of a brief distraction intervention on children's laboratory pain reactivity. Behav Modif 2003;27(2):217-32.
[16] Fanurik D, Zeltzer LK, Roberts MC, Blount RL. The relationship between children's coping styles and psychological interventions for cold pressor pain. Pain 1993;53(2):213-22.
[17] Reid GJ, Chambers CT, McGrath PJ, Finley GA. Coping with pain and surgery: children's and parents' perspectives. Int J Behav Med 1997;4(4):339-63.
[18] Lu Q, Zeltzer LK, Tsao JC, Kim SC, Turk N, Naliboff BD. Heart rate mediation of sex differences in pain tolerance in children. Pain 2005;118(1-2):185-93.
[19] Tsao JC, Myers CD, Craske MG, Bursch B, Kim SC, Zeltzer LK. Role of anticipatory anxiety and anxiety sensitivity in children's and adolescents' laboratory pain responses. J Pediatr Psychol 2004;29(5):379-88.
[20] Gragg RA, Rapoff MA, Danovsky MB, Lindsley CB, Varni JW, Waldron SA, et al. Assessing chronic musculoskeletal pain associated with rheumatic disease: further validation of the pediatric pain questionnaire. J Pediatr Psychol 1996;21(2):237-50.
[21] Hollingshead A. Two factor index of social position. New Haven, CT: Yale University, 1957.

[22] Johnson MH, Petrie SM. The effects of distraction on exercise and cold pressor tolerance for chronic low back pain sufferers. Pain 1997;69(1-2):43-8.

[23] Brewer B, and Karoly, P. Effects of attentional focusing on pain perception. Motivation Emotion 1989;13(3):193-203.

[24] Leventhal EA, Leventhal H, Shacham S, Easterling DV. Active coping reduces reports of pain from childbirth. J Consult Clin Psychol 1989;57(3):365-71.

[25] Ahles TA, Blanchard, E.B., and Leventhal, H. Cognitive control of pain: Attention to the sensory aspects of the cold pressor stimulus. Cogn Ther Res 1983;7:159-78.

[26] Piira T, Hayes B, Goodenough B, von Baeyer CL. Effects of attentional direction, age, and coping style on cold-pressor pain in children. Behav Res Ther 2006;44(6):835-48.

[27] McCaul KD, Haugtvedt C. Attention, distraction, and cold-pressor pain. J Pers Soc Psychol 1982;43(1):154-62.

[28] Roelofs J, Peters ML, van der Zijden M, Vlaeyen JW. Does fear of pain moderate the effects of sensory focusing and distraction on cold pressor pain in pain-free individuals? J Pain 2004;5(5):250-6.

[29] Hadjistavropoulos HD, Hadjistavropoulos T, Quine A. Health anxiety moderates the effects of distraction versus attention to pain. Behav Res Ther 2000;38(5):425-38.

[30] Fairhurst M, Wiech K, Dunckley P, Tracey I. Anticipatory brainstem activity predicts neural processing of pain in humans. Pain 2007;128(1-2):101-10.

V. Chronic pain

In: Children and Pain
Editors: P. Schofield and J. Merrick ISBN 978-1-60876-020-6

Chapter 7

How does chronic pain affect then lives of children?

Marcia L Meldrum, PhD*[*1], Jennie CI Tsao, PhD[2] and Lonnie K Zeltzer, MD[2]
[1]Department of History, University of California, Los Angeles
[2]Department of Pediatrics, David Geffen School of Medicine, University of California, Los Angeles, United States of America

Abstract

This chapter uses a mixed-methods approach to examine the impact of pain-associated functioning limitations on children's lives and the strategies they develop to try to continue functioning. Forty-five children ages 10-18 completed standardized questionnaires and participated in semistructured interviews prior to intake at a university-based tertiary clinic specializing in the treatment of pediatric chronic pain. All the children reported that pain limited their functioning in everyday activities and that these limitations caused them frustration and distress. Qualitative analysis identified three distinct functioning patterns or groups, which were designated as adaptive, passive and stressed. The groups did not differ significantly in demographics or clinical pain characteristics. Adaptive children continued to participate in many activities and were more likely to realize that focusing on pain would heighten their perception of pain. Children in this group reported more effective use of distraction and of other independently developed strategies to continue functioning. Passive children had given up most activities, tended to use passive distraction when in pain, and were more likely to feel isolated and different from peers. Stressed children described themselves as continuing to function, but were highly focused on their pain and the difficulties of living with it. The qualitative groupings were supported by quantitative findings that Stressed children reported a higher degree of social anxiety than did Passive children and were more likely than the other groups to report experiencing pain throughout the day. Finally,

* Correspondence: Marcia L. Meldrum, PhD, UCLA Pediatric Pain Study Group, 10940 Wilshire Boulevard, Suite 810, Los Angeles, CA 90024 United States. Tel: (310)-794-6290; E-mail: mlynnmel@earthlink.net

Adaptive children were rated by their parents as having better overall health compared to passive children.

Introduction

Chronic intractable non-malignant pain, with associated limitations in physical, academic, and social functioning, is a significant problem in children and adolescents. Several well-designed quantitative studies have shown that impaired functioning in children with chronic pain is strongly associated with psychosocial distress (1-3) and with lower quality of life (1,4-6), and that children with unexplained chronic pain often report significant dysfunctions in everyday activities (7). Although impaired functioning diminishes quality of life for children with chronic pain, we have relatively little research evidence regarding its prevalence and severity, why some children experience more limitations than others, how children and families cope with functioning limitations, and which treatment interventions are most successful in improving functioning (8).

Chronic non-malignant pain may persist for extended periods of time. Chronic idiopathic musculoskeletal pain was found in one report to persist in 59% of cases for up to nine years; the authors found the children to have pain and disability levels comparable to children with chronic juvenile arthritis (9). Hunfeld and colleagues in the Netherlands have shown that chronic benign pain may persist in 30-45% of cases for up to two years (10) and three years (11), although without increase in intensity or frequency. In the latter study, 42 adolescents described their functioning and coping skills in open-ended interviews, and identified ongoing problems with physical activity, mental concentration, social interaction, and psychological stress ("moodiness"), particularly with increased pain severity. Several of the children, however, had developed their own functioning strategies, including daily exercise and planning of daily routines: "…pain had become part of the daily lives of several adolescents, who structured their activities and sleeping hours to prevent aggravation of pain" (11).

A number of well-validated instruments have been developed for the assessment of functioning in children with chronic illness (for example, the Functional Disability Index (FDI) (12) and the Child Health Questionnaire (CHQ) (13,14)). Such quantitative self-report measures are excellent for comparing functioning levels between treatment groups, for tracking changes in groups over time, and for correlating functioning scores with scores on psychosocial and quality of life measures. But even well-validated quantitative instruments cannot fully assess the individual child's functioning choices and strategies, and his or perceived or real ability to continue to carry out specific real tasks in real-life situations. The items listed on the scale – "walking up the stairs" or "doing something with a friend" -- may or may not be those most important or most difficult for the child to accomplish daily. Moreover, quantitative self-report cannot fully describe the strategies children use to continue real-life functioning or what factors make a particular strategy most effective for a particular child.

This chapter reports on initial findings regarding the functioning limitations and strategies identified through mixed-methods analysis in a sample of 70 children reporting with chronic or recurrent pain to a university-based tertiary clinic. Both qualitative and quantitative data are examined to arrive at a better understanding of the impact of pain-associated functioning limitations on children's lives and the strategies they develop to try to continue functioning.

Our study

The participants were drawn from a larger sample of 175 children (122 girls, 69.7%) with a mean age of 14.2 years (SD = 2.4, range = 8-18 years), who presented for treatment at a multidisciplinary, tertiary clinic specializing in pediatric chronic pain between April 2003 and March 2005. The current study included 45 children (32 girls, 71.1%) with a mean age of 14.7 years (SD = 2.4, range = 10-18 years) who had completed videotaped oral history interviews prior to clinic intake. Ethnic composition for the present sample was: 64.4% Caucasian, 11.1% Latino, 2.2% African-American, 2.2% Asian American/Pacific Islander, 20.0% other (mixed race). Parents were mostly mothers (n = 36, 80.0%) with a mean age of 46.8 years (SD = 7.1, range = 32-67 years). Highest level of parent education was: high school diploma 5.3%, some college or associates degree 39.5%, college degree 26.3%, post-graduate degree 28.9%.

Among the 45 children in the current sample, presenting pain diagnoses were (note that percentages sum to more than 100% due to multiple pain diagnoses): 54.8% headaches (migraines; myofascial, vascular, tension, stress-related or other type of headaches), 45.2% myofascial pain (of any part of the body excluding headaches), 38.1% functional neurovisceral pain disorder (functional bowel, uterine, or bladder disorder), 14.3% complex regional pain syndrome, type 1 or type 2 (CRPS-I; CRPS-II) and 9.5% fibromyalgia. Multiple pain diagnoses were present in 52.4% (n = 22) of the sample. Children reported suffering pain for periods ranging from one month to "all my life": average duration of symptoms was 51.0 months (SD = 58.2, range = 1 – 215 months). All of them had seen at least one physician prior to referral to UCLA and the majority had seen three or more.

Qualitative procedures

The recruitment rate for the oral history component of the study was 57% of eligible children whose parents agreed to receive information about the study. The reasons most often given for non-participation were that the child was too ill to be interviewed or had too busy a schedule to allow time for the interview. Only two potential subjects objected to the videotaping of the interview. Three children who enrolled had to be excluded when there was not enough time for the interview to be scheduled prior to the clinic intake (as required by the study protocol). Although we cannot exclude the possibility of some selection bias, the children in the present sample did not differ from the full sample of 179 with respect to age, sex, race/ethnicity (Caucasian vs. non-Caucasian), which parent participated, parent age or parent education.

Fifty-one adolescents completed videotaped interviews between March 2003 and March 2005. Of these, six were withdrawn from the study: two cancelled the clinic intake appointment after the interview; two had to be excluded due to technical problems with the tape; one was withdrawn for medical reasons and one when an issue of domestic abuse arose during the interview. The remaining 45 are used in the current analysis.

Each child was interviewed at home, in his or her own room if possible. The interviewer was a trained graduate student who used a script which outlined the topics to be covered and provided suggested questions. However, interviewers were instructed to use probes and follow-up questions to elicit substantive answers and to allow the conversation to develop spontaneously at the child's own pace and level of interest. Interviews ranged in length from 45 to 135 minutes and were videotaped using a Sony camcorder. Although a few children were shy, most spoke quite freely and appeared comfortable with the taping. Several expressed satisfaction with the opportunity to speak freely to an interested neutral listener. The protocol called for the interview to be done privately and for the tapes not to be shown to parents.

Following the taping, DVD backups and audio tracks were made and the interviews transcribed by an experienced transcriber. Transcripts were reviewed for accuracy by the research team, proper names deleted and replaced by pseudonyms before analysis began. Transcripts were then coded using the N*6 coding program; codes were developed based on readings of the first set of transcripts and then continually reviewed and refined as the coding process developed. Using the coded interviews as guidelines, one researcher then conducted a grounded-theory analysis of the 45 initial interviews, reading each transcript several times, taking detailed notes on each interview, creating datasheets to track the recurrence of data and organize the data conceptually (15,16).

In some cases, where the transcriber had found it hard to understand the child, the videotape was reviewed to ensure the maximum accuracy possible. A second researcher independently tracked specific data items and the two analysts then compared these and resolved discrepancies. It should be emphasized that this was a preliminary analysis only, and that further refinements will emerge with the continuing work of the research team and with the transcription and analysis of the remaining 25 interviews and the 40 parent interviews conducted for this study.

Quantitative procedures

The procedure for administration of the quantitative measures has been described in detail previously (17,18). Briefly, prior to the initial clinic visit, two questionnaire packets, one for the child and one for a parent, were mailed to the home. Children and parents were instructed to complete the measures without consulting one another and to bring the packets with them to the initial clinic appointment. The quantitative measures assessed demographic and general health information including aspects of the child's pain, anxiety and functioning. Only measures relevant to the present investigation are discussed below.

Quantitative study measures

- Pain Intensity: A 10-cm Visual Analogue Scale (VAS) was used to represent a continuum from no pain to unendurable pain. The VAS is a reliable, valid, and widely used measure of pain intensity in children (19,20). This method measured the "usual" level of pain currently experienced by the child as reported by the child himself/herself.
- Child Health Questionnaire (CHQ PF50). The CHQ PF50 is a parent-completed instrument designed to measure the physical and psychosocial well-being of children with and without chronic conditions. The CHQ is one of the most widely used measures for children; it has sound psychometric properties (14). The CHQ PF50 contains 14 multi-item subscales: general health; physical functioning; role/social-physical; bodily pain; parent impact – time; parent impact – emotional; role/social – emotional; role/social – behavior; self-esteem; mental health; general behavior; family activities; family cohesion; change in health. In addition, the CHQ P50 contains a single item score for global health. This item assesses parents' rating of their overall child's health as excellent, very good, good, fair, or poor. For all CHQ scales, items are reversed when necessary and summed to attain raw scores which are then transformed into a 0-100 continuum. Higher scores on the CHQ scales indicate better functioning.
- Social Anxiety Scale for Children (SASC) Child report: The SASC is a 10-item child self-report measure of social anxiety. It has been shown to possess good psychometric properties, including internal consistency, test-retest reliability and construct validity (21). Factor analysis of the SASC supports a two-factor solution: Fear of Negative Evaluation (FNE) and Social Avoidance and Distress (SAD). FNE reflects concerns that other children will judge the respondent in a negative manner; SAD reflects social avoidance and social distress.
- Demographics and pain characteristics: Locally developed questionnaires completed by the parent assessed demographic information for children and parents including age, sex, race/ethnicity, and education. In addition, information regarding the part of the day children experience pain was assessed.
- Clinical Information: Information regarding pain diagnoses including duration of pain was derived from the patient's medical records via chart review. This information was recorded in the assessment portion of the initial evaluation report completed by the evaluating physician and recorded in the patient's medical chart.

Our findings

Qualitative findings

Functioning limitations stood out as the predominant theme in the set of 45 interviews. "It [the pain] keeps me from doing a lot of things I like." 35 of the 45 children (78%) stated that the major problem presented by the pain was that it had kept them out of school or from participating in a favorite activity. When asked how the pain made them feel, the children identified some 18 different emotions, including anger (14), depression (6) or sadness (7), fear (11), fatigue (10), worry (8), and acceptance or resignation (7), but the most frequently expressed emotion was frustration or annoyance (25) at the limitations they faced in normal functioning.

Children dealt with their limitations and frustrations in different ways. Through the process of inductive analysis and constant comparison, three recurrent patterns of behavior were identified, on the basis of which the children were divided into three groups, designated as Adaptive (A) (n = 13); Passive (P) (n = 13); and Stressed (S) (n = 19). The groups were based on these factors: children's school attendance; attitudes toward school attendance; participation in active (anything from softball to writing poetry) or passive (watching TV or resting) activities; primary coping behaviors when experiencing pain; attitudes toward activities dropped or abandoned because of pain; attitudes toward activities that were found difficult. Because the sample is small, not all observed differences can be quantified as statistically significant; but the common patterns in each group merit further study. Note that these patterns and differences were not determined by the researchers in advance, but were identified and assessed inductively through the process of constant comparison of the interview data presented by the children in their own words. Our qualitative analysis identified no major differences in the emotions expressed or kinds of stress factors identified by the three groups, but there were clear behavioral and attitudinal differences.

Four self-descriptive themes (see table 1) were identified recurrently in the interview data and tabulated independently of the factors considered in the analysis of functioning patterns. These were a) A sense of isolation and difference from peers. 53% of the children stated that they felt their pain separated them from their friends and classmates, who could not understand their experiences. For example, a 15 year old girl commented that "It's frustrating to see that it doesn't seem like they have to be as aware of like the inner workings of their body." b) A realization that expectation of, or attention to, pain increased the likelihood of feeling pain or increased its intensity. A significant minority (37%) of the children stated that they realized they were more likely to feel pain if they focused their attention on the pain site or asked themselves if they were feeling pain. c) Worries about the future. Although all the children stated concerns about whether the pain would prevent them from doing normal activities, slightly more than half (51%) talked about further worries that continuing pain that might prevent them from doing well in college, pursuing a career, or having the kind of life they had planned. d) Hiding the pain. More than half of the children (62%) stated that they tried to conceal the intensity and frequency of pain from parents, friends, and teachers, either because they didn't want others to worry about them or because they felt they could not understand.

Functioning groups: Patterns and differences

Adaptive children were the most able to continue to function. These children reported that they kept up school attendance, although they were sometimes forced to come home early if the pain was bad, and that they continued most activities. Half (6) reported having to give up a favorite activity, but all 13 discussed one or more activities in which they continued to participate. In coping with the pain, 4 stated they used medications, and 7 reported that they often just rested or slept; but all listed several distractions that helped them to ignore the pain and stay active. These children were more likely than those in the other two groups to realize that focusing on the pain would heighten their perception of pain, and less likely to report that they felt isolated or "different" from their peers (see table 1).

Passive children coped with pain by allowing it to take over their lives and limit their functioning. 11 of the 13 said that they coped by sleeping, "vegging", or "just curling up in a ball". Of the other two, one said that she stayed home and read, and the other that she relied on medication. Three others also mentioned medications. Only three in this group mentioned significant use of active distractions; while seven said they used passive distractions, such as watching TV or listening to music. Only three identified a favorite activity that they continued to participate in as much as possible. 10 of the 13 had missed significant amounts of school (two months or more), and in two cases, appeared to have abandoned the idea of ever returning. These children were more likely than those in the other two groups to report a sense of isolation from their peers.

Stressed children reported many types of coping behaviors and several made valiant attempts to continue functioning and to "fill the voids with happy things", but they were heavily focused on the pain and the limitations it imposed on them. Although four relied primarily on rest and medication to cope, most described using a combination of behaviors: these included active and passive distractions, changing eating or other habits, crying or focusing on the pain. All 19 described many limitations, while only five talked about a favorite activity they continued to pursue. Nine had missed significant amounts of school, and five were home-schooled or attending only a few classes. Although several stated that they tried to ignore or forget about the pain, children in this group were the least likely to state that they realized focusing on the pain might heighten their perception and discomfort. They were however the most likely to describe worries that the pain would continue and would interfere with their plans for college or a career (see table 1).

Finally, all 45 children reported some stress in their lives, usually from school work, concerns about grades, and/or peer relationships. The children in the Stressed group were slightly more likely than those in the other two groups to identify multiple sources of stress, but the difference could not be considered significant in this subsample. This topic will be reexamined in the larger sample.

Table 1. Self-descriptive themes and percentage reported by group

Theme	Full Sample (N=45)	Adaptive (N=13)	Passive (N=13)	Stressed (N=19)
Isolation from Peers	53%	23%	77%	53%
Realization that Focus on Pain May increase Pain Perception	37%	69%	38%	16%
Worries about Future	51%	38%	38%	68%
Hiding Pain from Others	62%	54%	69%	63%

Strategies

From our intensive review of the interview data, we concluded that simple listing of functions that the children could or could not perform, or found more or less difficult to do, was insufficient to explain the different levels of functioning. What emerged as a potentially more useful construct were the functioning strategies, combined cognitive and behavioral tools for dealing with pain, that were developed and used by the children. What may be most interesting about these strategies is that the children developed them independently: they had not been suggested by doctors, therapists, or parents, although it is likely that some of the children were imitating observed parent behavior. Three recurrent strategies were identified in this sample (individual children discussed below are identified by pseudonyms):

Getting on with things

Ignoring the pain and trying to keep going was the most common strategy discussed by children in both the Adaptive and Stressed groups. The difference was that the Adaptive group better incorporated the power of distraction into their strategy and focused on things besides the pain, as shown by these examples:

> "I'm keeping myself busy so I don't think about it," explains Andi, who is 16. When her headaches first developed, she stopped several of her favorite activities, and then started them again, one by one. When she is swimming, dancing or playing water polo, "I'm not thinking about, oh, my head hurts."

Thea is also 16; her love of music and singing impels her to go to school, even when she has headaches or abdominal pain. "I just know that if I go to school I get to sing, so I just try and focus on that…You can either let it control your life and just be in pain and not get anything done, or just be in pain and just move on, just work through it." Thea stated that she differed in this respect from her mother, who tended to stop all activity and rest when in pain.

Children in the Stressed group reported that their attempts to continue activities failed to distract them from the pain. Instead, their efforts caused them not only physical, but also emotional stress, and led to further impairment:

Marsha, who is 17, also says, "I just try to live normally and get on with it", but she is no longer playing basketball, which was her favorite activity. "I just kind of lost heart." She has missed a lot of school, but has kept up with the work, though she finds reading hard when her head aches, and she has continued swimming. Much of the time, though, she copes by sleeping or watching TV. She thinks of herself as "a strong person", but, having found "nothing takes the pain away completely," she is "just kind of losing faith that I'll get better."

Colin, also 17, has also been very active in sports and particularly loved water sports; for him, the ocean is "like Nirvana". He stated that his headaches sometimes stopped him from doing his school work or his much valued marine maintenance job, but not usually; "I just do whatever I need to do and produce." But trying to keep going when in pain makes him "real mean" and he "builds a wall" between himself and people he cares about; when he reaches this point, he retreats to "a quiet, dark room."

The differences in these children's accounts suggest that while "getting on with things" is a necessary strategic approach to continuing to function with pain, it may not always be sufficient. Several children in the Adaptive group also identified two other strategies which were not described by children in the other two groups (but which appear similar to those discussed by Hunfeld and colleagues (11)): planning ahead and body awareness.

Planning ahead

Cassie is 16 and involved in multiple activities at school, as well as using music and writing at home to take her mind off her fibromyalgia. She has found that "if I'm having fun, or if I'm doing something that's really important to me, then it's less severe and it's less a focus of my mind." But she also realized that, although she can usually "push through" physically, it's not always possible mentally, and she will become "easily aggravated or really petulant with people." Although she would prefer to be more spontaneous, therefore, she made a deliberate decision to organize her life to reduce stress and schedule more relaxing activities at the end of the day, when she would be tired. "I realized I had to like get an organizer and make sure I was really set and really organized and made sure that I didn't have anything really spontaneous to deal with, which kind of sucks....I find that it takes a lot of stress off to have a schedule and to know what you're doing and to be able to communicate that with other people."

Body awareness

Jade is 18 and uses music, reading, and painting successfully to distract herself from back pain: "I don't think the pain itself gets any different, but my awareness of it does." She has missed little school – "I'd rather go to school and be completely distracted and preoccupied" – and says she is "in charge" of her life, but thinks of the pain as a limiting factor. "What are other things that I could really enjoy doing, but I won't even let myself want to do them?" After she began practicing yoga, she was able to cope more effectively, she thinks, in that the practice "really changed the way that I look at my body and approach the pain. It definitely made me more aware of my body...how I hold myself and how I stand," and "much more observant of where I'm hurting and why." This awareness helps her when she tries to go to sleep at night and when she has to sit for long periods of time, both potential pain triggers.

Quantitative findings

Quantitative analyses comparing the three groups were conducted as follows. Oneway ANOVAs and chi-square tests for continuous and categorical data, respectively, were used to examine group differences across the study measures, i.e., the CHQ, SASC, demographics (sex, age, race/ethnicity, and parent education), pain characteristics (pain intensity, pain duration, type of pain diagnosis, presence of multiple pain diagnoses (yes/no), and parent report of the part of the day the child experienced pain). In the event of a significant omnibus F in the ANOVAs, post-hoc tests were conducted to specify which groups differed significantly. To test for differences based on race/ethnicity, children were classified as Caucasian vs. non-Caucasian. For each between-group comparison, children who had missing data were excluded from the analysis. A standard probability level of $p < .05$ was used to evaluate the results.

Demographic and pain characteristics

The demographic characteristics of the three groups are presented in table 2. The three groups did not differ on any of these demographic characteristics. The pain characteristics for the three groups are displayed in table 3. The groups differed significantly on the part of the day the child experienced pain according to parent report χ^2 (8) = 17.0, $p < .05$). As shown in table 3, nearly 65% of children in the Stressed group were reported to experience pain the entire day (24 hours), compared to roughly 12% in the Adaptive group and less than 30% in the Passive group. There were no other group differences in pain characteristics.

Table 2. Demographic data for the three study groups

	Adaptive		*Passive*		*Stressed*	
	M	*SD*	*M*	*SD*	*M*	*SD*
Mean Age (years)	14.7	2.8	14.3	1.8	14.8	2.6
	n	%	*N*	%	*N*	%
Gender Girls	10	76.9	10	76.9	12	63.2
Boys	3	23.1	3	23.1	7	36.8
Race/Ethnicity Caucasian	6	46.2	10	76.9	13	68.4
African-American	1	7.7	0	0	0	0
Latino/Hispanic	4	30.8	1	7.7	0	0
Asian-American/Pacific Islander	0	0	1	7.7	0	0
Other	2	15.4	1	7.7	6	31.6
Parent Education						
High School diploma	0	0	0	0	2	11.1
Some college/Associate's degree	2	22.2	6	54.5	7	38.9
College degree	4	44.4	2	18.2	4	22.2
Post-graduate degree	3	33.3	3	27.3	5	27.8

Table 3. Descriptive data on pain characteristics for the three study groups

	Adaptive		*Passive*		*Stressed*	
	N	%	*n*	%	*n*	%
Pain Diagnosis						
Headaches	7	53.8	6	50.0	10	58.8
Myofascial	5	38.5	6	50.0	8	47.1
FNPD	4	30.8	7	58.3	5	29.4
CRPS	2	15.4	2	16.7	2	10.5
Fibromyalgia	1	7.7	0	0	3	17.6
Multiple Pain Diagnosis (yes)	4	30.8	9	75.0	9	52.9
Pain Duration	*Months*	*SD*	*Months*	*SD*	*Months*	*SD*
	41.1	44.2	47.4	50.7	60.9	72.5
Pain Intensity	*Mean*	*SD*	*Mean*	*SD*	*Mean*	*SD*
	5.8	1.4	5.7	2.1	6.6	1.6

	Adaptive		*Passive*		*Stressed*	
Part of the day pain is experienced						
Extremely small (< 1 hour)	2	25.0	0	0	0	0
Small (1-8 hours)	1	12.5	3	27.3	1	5.9
Almost half day (9-14 hours)	0	0	2	18.2	2	11.8
Most of the day (15-23 hours)	4	50.0	3	27.3	3	17.6
Entire day (24 hours)	1	12.5	3	27.3	11	64.7

Note: Frequencies for pain diagnoses sum to more than 100% due to multiple pain diagnoses. FNPD = functional neurovisceral pain disorder; CPRS = complex regional pain syndrome, type 1 or type 2; Pain intensity: range = 0 -10.

Global health and social functioning

On the CHQ, parent ratings of the child's global health differed significantly across the groups ($F(2,35) = 3.48$, $p < .05$). Post-hoc tests revealed that the Adaptive group (M = 65.6; SD = 32.2) scored higher than the Passive group (M = 28.2; SD = 36.0), indicating better perceived global health in the former group. This finding offers confirmation from the parent's perspective that the Adaptive group was perceived as functioning better than the Passive group. The Stressed group (M = 35.8; SD = 32.1) did not differ from the other two groups. There were no other group differences on the CHQ.

For the SASC total scores, there was a significant difference among the groups ($F(2,34) = 3.48$, $p < .05$). Post-hoc tests indicated that the Stressed group (M = 9.0; SD = 4.9) reported higher scores than the Passive group (M = 4.3; SD = 2.5), indicating higher overall social anxiety in the former compared to the latter group. The Adaptive group (M = 5.9; SD = 3.8) did not differ from the other two groups. Analysis comparing the SASC subscales revealed a significant group difference for the FNE subscale ($F(2,34) = 4.74$, $p < .05$) but no such difference for the SAD subscale. Post-hoc tests indicated that the Stressed group (M = 5.7; SD = 4.1) scored higher than the Passive group (M = 2.5; SD = 2.0) on the FNE subscale indicating higher fear of negative evaluation in the former group; the Adaptive group (M = 3.7; SD = 2.8) did not differ from the other two groups.

Discussion

Qualitative analysis of interviews with 45 children prior to clinic intake identified three well-differentiated functioning patterns, which were designated as Adaptive, Stressed, and Passive. The qualitative analysis found clear behavioral and attitudinal differences between the groups in school attendance, activity participation, and coping behaviors. Baseline quantitative analysis (see tables 2 and 3 below) identified no significant differences between the three groups of children in demographic factors, or reported pain intensity or duration; however, the Stressed children reported higher overall social anxiety than the children in the Passive group, and they were the most likely of the three groups to report experiencing pain throughout the entire day (see table 3). As displayed in table 3, nearly 65% of Stressed children reported experiencing pain the entire day compared to approximately 12% of children in the Adaptive group and roughly 27% of children in the Passive group. Our quantitative analyses also revealed significant differences in parental perceptions of children's global health. The Adaptive group were rated by parents as being in better overall health compared the children in the Passive group; although parents of children in the Stressed group also rated their children's global health as being worse than that of the Adaptive group, this difference was not statistically significant.

Qualitative analyses further revealed that the three groups showed significant differences in self-descriptive themes independently derived from the interview data: the Adaptive group was more likely to be aware that focusing on pain increased the likelihood of pain perception; the Passive group was more likely to report a sense of isolation and difference from peers; and the Stressed group was more likely to report that they were worried about the impact of pain on their future.

Although all 45 children in this sample reported functioning limitations due to chronic pain, Adaptive children appeared to present with a more effective approach to functioning than the Stressed or Passive children. One possible explanation is that the Adaptive children have developed more effective functioning strategies. Although both Adaptive and Stressed children stated that they tried to "get on with things", the Adaptive children were more able to use favorite activities as positive distractions from the pain. They also had developed additional strategies to help them function, of which two, "planning ahead" and "body awareness", are discussed above.

It should not be minimized that pain intensity levels were comparable for all three groups, Adaptive, Passive, and Stressed, and that all of the children in our sample were sufficiently bothered by pain to seek care at a tertiary clinic specializing in pediatric pain. What this preliminary analysis indicates is that, for all three groups, the major impact of pain was that it limited their ability to do the things they wanted to do; and that each child had adapted an individual pattern of cognitions and behaviors that either promoted or impaired their ability to continue functioning. Although standard quantitative self-report measures did not reveal a great many differences associated with these patterns, qualitative analysis was able to identify and characterize three groups with distinct attitudinal and behavioral differences and to present a rich and complex description of the children's functioning.

At least one subset of the sample, the Adaptive group, had managed to "normalize" a life with chronic pain to some degree, in a manner similar to that described in children with other chronic diseases (22,23); but they remained conscious of it as a continuing source of distress and limitation, one that they had to continue to deal with in their efforts to remain normal. While it seems a reasonable inference that children in the Passive and Stressed groups might function better if they were more Adaptive, they would in all probability still have pain.

The questions that suggest themselves at this point, therefore, are, first, are these strategic approaches at baseline in any way associated with more positive pain and functioning outcomes following changes in treatment and management recommended at a tertiary clinic? Second, will some children become more Adaptive during treatment, and will they then show more positive outcomes than those who become, or remain, Passive or Stressed? Third, if further evidence supports the finding that a number of children are able to develop effective functioning strategies on their own, are there ways in which clinicians can promote better strategies in children who are functioning less well?

These questions will be considered in our further analysis of this sample of 45 children at six-month follow-up and of the full sample of 70 children who participated in this study between 2003 and 2006.

Cognitive-behavioral therapy is certainly one therapeutic option that may be appropriate here and has been shown to benefit children and adolescents with chronic pain (24,25). However, this option is not available, affordable, or acceptable to every family. Inasmuch as some children demonstrate individual patterns of skills that have helped them cope with pain, the possibility of developing and promoting these skills in other children should be explored.

Further research along these lines is also merited, particularly longitudinal studies which follow children with chronic pain through college and young adulthood. The long-term impact of pain and associated functioning impairment is not known. Nor is it clear that functioning skills developed in adolescence are transferable to later life. Hunfeld and colleagues raise the question that the strategic approaches reported in their study (11) may only work well for adolescents, who are protected from the daily responsibilities and stresses of having to make a living, manage their own homes, and so forth, faced by adults. Better answers to all these questions are needed in order to help the many young people whose lives are diminished by chronic pain.

Acknowledgments

This research was supported by NIMH grant R01 MH 063779 (PI Margaret C. Jacob) and by a seed grant from the Mayday Fund. The invaluable suggestions, advice, and help of Ignasi Clemente, the administrative assistance of Edward Curnen, and the interviewing, coding, and transcription work of Mara Buchbinder, Arianne Gaetano, Reynal Guillen, Ryan Hodgkinson, Marian Katz, Tanya Stivers, and Suzanne Walter are gratefully acknowledged.

References

[1] Bandell-Hoekstra IENG, Abu-Saad HH, Passchier J, Frederiks CAM, Feron FJM, Knipschild P. Coping and quality of life in relation to headaches in Dutch schoolchildren. Eur J Pain 2002;6: 315-21.

[2] Kashikar-Zuck S, Goldschneider KR, Powers SW, Vaught MH, Hershey AD. Depression and functional disability in chronic pediatric pain. Clin J Pain 2001;17: 341-9.

[3] Reid GJ, Lang BA, McGrath PJ. Primary juvenile fibromyalgia: Psychological adjustment, family functioning, coping, and functional disability. Arthritis Rheumatism 1997;40: 752-60.

[4] Hunfeld JA, Perquin CW, Duivenvoorden HJ, Hazebroek-Kampschreur AAJM, Passchier J, van Suijlekom-Smit LWA, van der Wouden JC. Chronic pain and its impact on quality of life in adolescents and their families. J Pediatr Psychol 2001;26:145-53.

[5] Nodari E, Battistella PA, Naccarella C, Vidi M. Quality of life in young Italian patients with primary headache. Headache 2002;42: 268-74.

[6] Powers SW, Patton SR, Hommel KA, Hershey AD: Quality of life in childhood migraines: clinical impact and comparison with other childhood illnesses. Pediatrics 2003; 112: e1-5.
[7] Konijnenberg AY, Uiterwaal CSPM, Kimpen JLL, van der Hoeven J, Buitelaar JK, de Graeff-Meeder ER. Children with unexplained chronic pain: Substantial impairment in everyday life. Arch Dis Childhood 2005;90: 680-6.
[8] Palermo TM. Impact of recurrent and chronic pain on child and family daily functioning: A critical review of the literature. J Dev Behav Pediatrics 2000;21:58-69.
[9] Aasland A, Flato B, Vandvik IH. Psychosocial factors in children with idiopathic musculoskeletal pain: A prospective, longitudinal study. Acta Paediatr 1997;86:740-6.
[10] Perquin CW, Hunfeld JA, Hazebroek-Kampschreur AAJM, van Suijlekom-Smith LWA, Passchier J, Koes BW, van der Wouden JC. The natural course of chronic benign pain in childhood and adolescence: A two-year population-based follow-up study. Eur J Pain 2003;7:551-9.
[11] Hunfeld JA, Perquin CW, Bertina W, Hazebroek-Kampschreur AlAJM, van Suijlekom-Smith LWA, Koes BW, van der Wouden JC, Passchier J. Stability of pain parameters and pain-related quality of life in adolescents with persistent pain: A three-year follow-up. Clin J Pain 2002;18:99-106.
[12] Walker LS, Greene JW. The functional disability inventory: Measuring a neglected dimension of child health status. J Pediatr Psychol 1991;6:39-58.
[13] Asmussen L, Olson LM, Grant EN, Landgraf JM, Fagan J, Weiss KB. Use of the child health questionnaire in a sample of moderate and low-income inner-city children with asthma. Am J Resp Critical Care Med 2000;162:1215-21.
[14] Landgraf JM, Abetz L, Ware JE. The CHQ: A user's manual. 2nd printing. Boston, MA: Health Institute, 1999.
[15] Glaser BG. Strauss AL. The discovery of grounded theory: Strategies for qualitative research. Chicago: Aldine, 1967.
[16] Charmaz K. "Discovering" chronic illness: Using grounded theory. Soc Sci Med 1990;30:1161-72.
[17] Bursch B, Tsao JCI, Meldrum M, Zeltzer LK. Preliminary validation of a self-efficacy scale for child functioning despite chronic pain (child and parent versions). Pain 2006;125:35-42.
[18] Tsao JCI, Meldrum M, Bursch B, Jacob MC, Kim SC, Zeltzer LK. Treatment expectations for CAM interventions in pediatric chronic pain patients and their parents. Evidence-Based Compl Alternative Med 2005;2:521-7.
[19] McGrath PJ. There is more to pain measurement in children than "ouch". Can Psychol 1996;37:63-75.
[20] Varni J W, Walco GA, Katz ER. Assessment and management of chronic and recurrent pain in children with chronic diseases. Pediatrician 1989;16:56-63.
[21] La Greca AM, Dandes SK, Wick P, Shaw K. Development of the social anxiety scale for children: Reliability and concurrent validity. J Clin Child Psychol 1998;17: 84-91.
[22] Admi H. Growing up with a chronic health condition: A model of an ordinary lifestyle. Qual Health Res 1996;6:163-83.
[23] Stewart JL. Getting used to it: Children finding the ordinary and routine in the uncertain context of cancer. Qual Health Res 2003;13: 394-407.
[24] Degotardi PJ, Klass ES, Rosenberg BS, Fox DG, Gallelli KA, Gottlieb BS. Development and evaluation of a cognitive-behavioral intervention for juvenile fibromyalgia. J Pediatr Psychol 2006;31: 714-23.
[25] Eccleston C, Malleson PM, Clinch J, Connell H, Sourbut C. Chronic pain in adolescents: Evaluation of a programme of interdisciplinary cognitive behaviour therapy. Arch Dis Childhood 2003;88:881-5.

In: Children and Pain
Editors: P. Schofield and J. Merrick
ISBN 978-1-60876-020-6

Chapter 8

The needs of adolescents with chronic pain

Paula Forgeron**, RN, MN and Patrick J McGrath, OC, PhD, FRSC
Pediatric Complex Pain Management Team and IWK Health Centre,
Dalhousie University, Halifax, Nova Scotia, Canada

Abstract

In this chapter we used a focus group interview to explore the self-identified needs of adolescents living with chronic pain. Nineteen youth, who receive care through the Chronic Pain Clinic at a tertiary care children's hospital were invited to participate. Six youth, age 13-17years, consented to participate. The discussions were transcribed verbatim and thematic analysis was conducted. Two major themes emerged from the data; struggling to be normal, and dealing with the pain. Participants view themselves as different and unhealthy compared to their peers. Health is seen as "being normal"; "able to do whatever you want". Distraction was the primary strategy for coping with pain. Friends were seen as essential to well being but understanding was limited. Half of the participants felt that peers who had pain would provide a major source of support. Those not in favour of this support cited the idiosyncratic nature of pain. School was uniformly identified as the greatest source of stress. The thought of transition to adult care was overwhelming. They were unsure what skills they needed in order to transition, and asserted they were not ready to transition to adult service.

Introduction

Adolescents with chronic pain face many challenges; they suffer from a disease process that is not well understood, has an uncertain illness trajectory, and is not usually accompanied by

* Correspondence: Paula Forgeron, RN, MN, Clinical Nurse Specialist, Pediatric Complex Pain Management Team, IWK Health Centre, 5850/5980 University Avenue, POBox 9700, Halifax, Nova Scotia, B3K 6R8, Canada. Tel: (902) 470-6350; Fax (902) 470-7911; E-mail: pforgero@dal.ca

obvious physical signs. Hence many teens face disbelief from friends, family, and health professionals (1,2). In addition, although up to 25% of children and or adolescents may develop chronic pain at some point in their childhood (3,4), most adolescents with chronic pain feel isolated as they do not have peers with a similar chronic pain experience (1,2). As a result, youth with chronic pain must learn ways to cope with these many challenges. We could not find any studies that identified what youth believe their needs to be. Understanding the self-identified needs of youth with chronic pain will assist in designing ways to meet these needs.

Our qualitative study captured what youth identified as helpful in coping with chronic pain and which areas of their lives they needed help. Youth identified that they struggled with being the same as their peers. Despite finding ways to cope with pain, issues such as academic workload, talking to friends, dealing with peers who were not friends, and preparing to transition to adult services were challenging.

Chronic pain in children and adolescents results from "a dynamic integration of biological processes, psychological factors, and sociocultural context considered within a developmental trajectory" (5). Coping is a process of changing behavioral and cognitive efforts to manage specific external and/or internal demands that an individual appraises as taxing or beyond their resources (6). Hence coping is contextually based, and therefore an understanding of coping would be enhanced by examining the description of thoughts and actions that take place in stressful encounters (6). Pain also changes over time and may depend on the context. Given the variable nature of coping and pain we believe understanding what is needed to improve pain coping is embedded in the experiences of those living with pain.

Our study

We used a fundamental qualitative approach (7) to provide a descriptive analysis of the data to discover and understanding the phenomena from the perspective of the specific population (8). A focus group was used to elicit the experiences and needs of the adolescents with chronic pain. Interactions among participants can generate more in-depth information than one could obtain in a survey (9), and provides an opportunity to clarify agreement, or disagreement within the group, by observing body language, as well as, listening to the dialogue among participants as they respond to questions and comments (10). The study took place at the only pediatric chronic pain clinic for the Maritime Provinces in Canada.

Participants

A purposeful sample was obtained by inviting all current eligible adolescent patients from the pediatric chronic pain clinic to participate. The medical director of the clinic endorsed the study and mailed letters to the patients. This letter included a brief description of the study along with the contact information of the researchers; interested patients were instructed to contact the researchers directly.

Eligible patients between the ages of 12-18 years of age who spoke English fluently were invited to participate. Youth with cognitive impairments or cancer pain were excluded. The letter announcing the study was sent to 19 eligible youth. Eight called to receive consent packages. Two of these patients were unable to participate due to prior commitments on the day of the focus group. Six youth participated in the focus group. Travel expenses were reimbursed for participants.

Five of the six participants were female and ranged in age from 13 to 18 years. Participants were in grade 8 to 12, which was appropriate for their age. They were all from Caucasian middle-class socioeconomic families and lived at home with both parents.

Data collection

A self-administered eleven-item demographic questionnaire was completed prior to the focus group discussion. A semi-structured interview guide was used to keep the discussion flowing. The discussion was audiotaped and transcribed verbatim. Refreshments were provided. The adolescents had never met prior to the focus group so the session started with introductions, followed by a review of the rationale for the focus group, and a discussion on respecting everyone's comments and experiences. Confidentiality was reviewed. Participants were reassured that their would be no names or identifying features attached to their comments and quotes in discussions, papers and presentations.

The youth were shy at first but opened up to sharing their experiences. Often the participants shared experiences with each other as opposed to answering the questions posed by the facilitator. All participants contributed to the discussion. No adolescents left or declined to answer any of the questions.

Data analysis

The focus group discussion was thematically analyzed. Open coding (11) was conducted on the transcripts by the first author by reading the entirety of the transcript several times to gain an impression of the overall experiences of the participants. A list of identified labels was developed from the data during this process and the categorizing scheme was continually refined during analysis. The data were then clustered under the established category headings and themes identified. Validity of the themes was determined through constant comparison, which has been described as the distribution of data into specific categories based on whether the contents "look-alike" or "feel-alike" until all data are accounted for (12).

Our findings

The participants had been attending the pain clinic for over a year and had experienced pain from 13 months to 10 years. Pain location varied and included pelvic area, shoulders, neck, back, hands, feet, left knee, and stomach. Two participants had pain in only one location and one participant had short periods of no pain. All participants had pain on daily basis, ranging from 3-9/10 on a 0 to 10 scale, with exacerbations escalating between 6-10/10. Despite individual difference, they all experienced pain that interfered with daily life and prevented them from participating in their favorite activities and sports with school absences between 2 to 13 days/month. Five of the participants were on medication and the sixth had trials of various medications. All participants received instruction on psychological pain management techniques by the pediatric pain psychologist, and all but one received physiotherapy.

There were two over-riding themes that emerged from the focus group data; "Struggling to be Normal" and "Dealing with the Pain". These themes transcended the stories that the adolescents shared and shed light on the needs of these adolescents to enhance coping.

Struggling to be normal

All of the participants told stories of wanting to be like their peers, who they viewed as normal. Pain interrupted their ability to function to the extent that they felt abnormal. Their pain caused them to take medications, attend various appointments, miss out on activities, or be absent from school, which only served to remind them that their lives were deeply altered and different from their peers. Several sub themes emerged in their struggle to be normal.

Healthy is being normal

Overall the participants did not see themselves as healthy at the time of the focus group. From their definitions, health was synonymous with being normal and is exemplified in this female participant's quote "The key word is normal. You have to be able to feel like you're normal and not outside of like everyone else." The salient characteristic of being healthy centered on activity. As the male in the group explained, " I think it [health] means that you can do whatever you want". Pain was not only seen as preventing engagement in activities but also restricting the amount of time they had for activities by attending to the demands of treatment. "Like, most 17 year olds don't go to physiotherapy 3, 4, 5 times a week, and you know, go to the pain clinic. Most normal teenagers don't do that. I am far from the norm—far, far from the norm" (female participant). These statements on health illustrate that the adolescents viewed health through the lens of normal adolescent behavior, not physiologic impairments. Even for the two adolescents who had other chronic illnesses, it was the restrictions caused by their pain that made them feel unhealthy.

Trying to be normal at school

Although they all wanted to be seen as normal, and did not want attention drawn to themselves in the classroom, each voiced a need to have modifications to their academic requirements and all were stressed and frustrated when modifications were not offered. One of the participants started the discussion about school by saying, "school is a killer". This comment was received with laughter, sighs of understanding, and agreement by nodding of heads from others. They struggled academically because of their pain and this struggle interfered dramatically with their desire to be normal. Trying to keep up marks was difficult due to the cognitive effects of pain, which was exacerbated by the amount of school absence. As one participants comment, "When I was trying to make the honor role last year it [pain] was bad, like before every test I was like I'm gonna puke." Another noted that "Grade eleven sucks, I can usually concentrate when I am there but when I miss like a week of chemistry [due to pain], I'm lost."

Despite not wanting to differ from their peers, they all acknowledged that this was impractical at times. Being absent from school, needing to leave class, getting up to stretch, or inability to participate in physical education class were impossible to hide. However, for a few this was made worse by teachers who were described as fussing over them, asking in class if they were OK, or not getting upset with their behavior when other pupils would have been disciplined for the same action. These situations increased their unease with standing out. Not all the participants experienced the 'over caring' teachers. Most struggled with teachers not providing agreed upon accommodations for their pain. This was perceived as disbelief from their teachers. As one adolescent shared, "Like if I'm sick then too bad—oh well, they don't care. They say like that's your problem." This was very problematic for this young woman who was in her final year of high school and trying to attain the necessary grades to be accepted into university. She felt that her marks had dropped as a result of missed class time and that her teachers did not want to assist her in obtaining the missed content. Others voiced similar experiences resulting in an increase in stress related pain, a decrease in marks, and, for some, disengagement from academic pursuits.

One of the youth said that he did not study for tests anymore as he would get "pissed off because half of the things [notes] I don't have", the result of not receiving information or help for missed content. Another participant empathized and stated that there is "no sense in studying if you don't have the stuff." Even when they try to find the material for themselves one said, "You have to write all these notes from your friends and that's going to take even longer and you're going to get less time to study".

Another noted, "it's frustrating because you know you can, like, make a certain mark and usually you do really awesome and then with pain sometimes you can't finish this or you can't finish that. You are capable of so much more but you're kind of screwed." Although all of the participants shared stories of struggles at school, two of the participants shared how things had improved once their teachers understood, or, at least, made agreed upon accommodations. Provision of notes, decreased workload, and flexible assignment and test dates were essential components of supportive academic accommodations. Even though other factors, such as absences from school and being excused from physical education, still made them stand out as different, these two adolescents now felt positive about their academic abilities.

Relating to peers and society interferes with being normal

There was a unanimous agreement that relating to peers who were not friends and society in general reminded them that they were different and they struggled with how to relate. This occurred everywhere in their communities: at the grocery store, pharmacy, church, group activities, and school. They spoke of these interactions as different from those with their teachers and friends, as they were willing to share some of their health history with teachers and friends to gain their support and understanding. The participants shared stories of relative strangers asking them personal health questions. One participant explained, "people that you don't even talk to or even know, they just come up and ask you how you are doing." Some of these interactions occurred after discharge from hospital but other interactions occurred for no apparent reason. Some random girl walked up like, I was in the hospital three years ago and she was like are you still sick? I hadn't been in the hospital for like three years and she asks are you better yet? I never talk to her; I don't know how the hell she knew I was ever in the hospital. I was like I've been out of the hospital for like three years and she was like oh, I didn't know that. She then asked me what's wrong with you? I just didn't want to talk to her and I just walked away and she was swearing at me and stuff. (male participant)

Another participant recounted her first outing after being in hospital for her pain. She went to the pharmacy with her mother and felt as though everyone in the pharmacy came up and asked her what was wrong with her. Although she believed most were trying to show concern the questioning was overwhelming and left her wanting to leave and remembered saying, "Mom, take me home because I don't want to be around anyone." The other participants revealed similar experiences and as one adolescent said, "Yeah, like they're always asking and I really hate it because I don't want to tell the whole world that I'm sick [in pain]. I just want to be back to normal, a normal teenager living my life without everyone having to know that I'm sick [in pain]".

These interactions reminded them that they were different than their peers, as virtual strangers did not ask other adolescents such personal questions. In addition, not only were these interactions an invasion of their privacy they resulted in other negative experiences. As noted in one of the exchanges the adolescent was subjected to cursing when he ignored a girl's questions. Another participant explained how people pitied her. "A lot of people give me pity and that's not something I want. I don't want to be pitied or treated any different than anyone else just because of what's going on." All of participants expressed that they did not want to have to explain their pain condition to everyone. They had already experienced disbelief from people they either knew or trusted, such as health care professionals, and desired privacy from strangers.

Dealing with the pain

Dealing with the pain was a daily occurrence. Some felt that the pain had a life of its own, while others verbalized a more cavalier attitude towards their pain, stating that it was "not ruling their life". Regardless of their professed belief they shared stories that illustrated that their pain did dictate aspects of their lives. Yet, their stories were also filled with courage and a desire to move forward.

Management strategies

The participants found strategies to deal with their pain but none had found these to be successful in all situations or all the time. All but one of the participants took analgesics to help manage their pain. Although generally helpful, these medications were not useful during exacerbations. As one participant explained, "When it [the pain] hits a certain level then its gonna go its own path" and the medications were no longer very effective.

Activity was a challenge for each of the group but in varying degrees. One of the female participants commented, "I am active to the degree that I can be without being in pain." Although the concept of pacing had been reviewed, they found it difficult to pace their activities incorporate pacing into their lives, and unconvinced of the benefit. One girl clarified the difficulties with pacing by saying "I can't really help [by pacing activity], because you don't know when it [the pain] is going to come, it comes from anything." However, another stated "I can't pack it in because I get really, really tired and tired just doesn't help the pain and then this whole spiral effect starts to happen." So, for all but one participant they had fun when they felt good. As one girl noted, she did activities even if it resulted in increased pain, "I went to the movies the other night and I said I know I'm going to hurt [as I was overdoing it] but I really wanted to go to the movies." Dealing with increased pain was seen as a necessary consequence of engaging in activities: "There is a level of pain that like goes up if I do certain things, but I know it is going to go back to normal pain, so like she was saying, I do like to get out and do stuff, like remain sane."

The one strategy that they all used and agreed was most effective after their medication was distraction. As one stated, "Distraction is my main thing. Anything to get my mind off of it." In most instances the participants had found unique ways to distract themselves. They shared their best distraction strategies, and these ranged from playing piano, listening to music, going for run, using the computer, going to a tanning bed, to having their friends tell them stories while they were in school. One girl described distraction while at school, "If I'm at school and get an episode [of pain] I'm like OK, talk and talk with my friend and I'm focusing on her and not what's going on with my pain."

Relating to friends

Pain complicated the adolescents' relationships with their friends. Friends' disbelief and, or, inability to grasp the impact of pain was a common and distressing experience. As one participant revealed, "they don't really understand when you say I can't go because I'm going to end up getting sick." Although some said it was helpful to talk to their friends about the frustrations of living with pain this was not true all the time, or, for all participants. One shared that her friends are "useless from a pain point of view". None of the participants had a visible abnormality to account for their pain and believed that this contributed to the disbelief they encounter from friends and society. This was exemplified by this participant's account.

They all [my friends] think that I'm full of it, they all think that I don't have any pain and uh, that I must be making it up because I don't take medication, because I refuse to. But they don't see the side effects. The side effects that hit me are like I sit on my kitchen floor because my room is spinning. Like it's horrible and they thinking I'm making it up.

Despite the struggles with friends the participants were quick to excuse their friends' lack of understanding. One participant explained that, "friends are helpful to a point but they can't fully understand because they haven't gone through it." Trying to explain everything to their friends became tiring and was reported at times to increase confusion amongst their friends. " Well like, the first year I had pain and at the hospital and stuff that was the only time we ever talked about where I was and what happened. But they did not really understand they just wanted to know how much it hurt and can you still play basketball? "(male participant).

Three participants in the group had a friend who also struggled with a health condition; one of these three had a friend with chronic pain. These friendships were described as being different from their other friends. "One best friend, she's like my sister she like lives at our house. She kind of gets what it's like to be different. She has diabetes and kidney disease so she knows what it's like to have to miss school for appointments and such".

The participant who had a chronic pain friend described the relationship as helpful in the following way. "Oh my gosh, she has made a world of difference in my life. I found talking with her helped. I could tell her anything. I didn't think it would be that awesome or great to have someone with pain to talk to, [but] that's what really helps me—not feeling so alone".

A few of the participants expressed that it would be "cool to meet someone who has close to the same thing" but others were skeptical of finding such a person, as they believed that their pain was unique and rare. Other reasons for not being keen on the idea of a pain buddy included not wanting to be reminded of their pain by talking about it or talking with strangers about their condition. It is unclear if some of these participants felt that meeting someone else with pain would once again make them feel abnormal, as healthy peers do not have this sort of 'special' friend.

Transitioning—not yet

When transitioning to adult care was introduced most of the participants expressed discomfort with the idea. All believed that one should be an adult before moving to adult care facilities and none of them felt that they were adults yet. There was an acknowledgement from the older participants that they felt too old for a pediatric hospital but too young for an adult hospital. As one noted "Not until I am 18 years old, 20 is technically an adult. Like I am not an adult when I am 16, I would be still a teenager in an adult hospital." Most others agreed with this statement and included criteria such as being out of high school and able to drive themselves to appointments as signs of adulthood. One suggested, "they should give you a choice of when you want to leave, but the limit would be like 20. So, if you're ready to leave when you're 16 then you can". The other participants agreed that they should have more say in when to transition.

The participants cited other discomforts with transitioning. They did not look forward to getting to know new health professionals and having to tell their story again. They voiced concerns over what the adult health care professionals would be like, in particular, would they be believed. This concern was exemplified by one participant who had been seen in an adult clinic for a second opinion, "Like the way they worded things, like they were almost trying to trick you to like thinking like their way, and I'm like no [I really have pain]."

None of the participants cited self-advocacy, or self-management skills as necessary to interact successfully in an adult system. Parents still attended appointments, called for the youth's prescription renewals, and were responsible to contact health professionals when questions arose. Only one had independently called to ask questions or discuss her needs with the members of the pain care team. When asked if these skills were required before transitioning they agreed but were surprised that their parents' involvement in their care might change when they were transitioned. The group felt that it would be important to start taking more ownership of their care but wanted this to evolve slowly, such as attending a portion of their appointments by themselves.

The adolescents were concerned about their futures; would pain still be present, would it decrease, would they be able to manage and pursue their dreams. Transitioning to adult care was yet another challenge that they had to mount in dealing with pain. They spoke of the impending event with great reservation and viewed the physical environment as void of caring. As one of the participants noted, "Yeah, but the bad thing about the adult care system is that there are so many colours here it makes you feel happier but in there [adult clinic] it is just white".

Discussion

Our research identified several needs of this group of adolescents suffering with chronic pain. They view themselves as unhealthy and different compared to their peers. Although other studies (1, 2) have identified that adolescents with chronic pain feel isolated from their peers at times, the participants in this study spoke of struggles that encompassed more than feelings of isolation. Their stories shed light on how deeply they viewed themselves as different. They felt alienated from the mainstream and did not see themselves as being normal members of society. They even described health as being normal. However, part of their definition of health, being able to engage in activities that they want, is similar to that found that in other studies with children and adolescents (13, 14).

Although viewing themselves as different they did not want to be seen as different, or sick, and tried to do what they could to appear similar to peers. This desire to not be seen as sick is not unique to adolescents with chronic pain (15). Despite not wanting to appear sick there were constant reminders that they were different. Their pain complicated conversations with friends and resulted, at times, in self-imposed isolation to avoid personal questions. Lazrus (6) asserted, that when an individual believes little or nothing can be done the emphasis is apt to be placed on emotion-focused coping processes, whereas when the situation is believed to be changeable problem-focused approaches are apt to prevail. It is not known if these adolescents would have engage more fully with others if they thought differently about the situation or felt competent in their skill to discuss their pain with others.

Perceived disbelief among teachers and non-friend peers contributed to sources of stress at school. Trying to catch up on missed information and teach themselves concepts while dealing with the cognitive effects of pain, increased stress related pain. These adolescents cited accommodations as essential to achieve academic success and prevent them from falling behind their peers. Teachers' willingness to make accommodations were viewed as an acknowledgement that their pain was real, otherwise they felt punished for their condition. Despite being at different stages of adolescence and illness trajectory they all agreed that a problem-focused coping strategy including the provision of notes, flexible timelines, and a decreased workload were needed and that a more active involvement by health care professionals helped secure these accommodations. The individuality of this coping process was in the degree of accommodation required.

Greco, Freeman, and Dufton (16) found that children and adolescents with undiagnosed abdominal pain were subject to increases in overt and relational victimization, while Kashikar-Zuck et al (17) discovered that youth with fibromyalgia are not as likable compared to normative classmates. Comparatively, the adolescents in this study described being misunderstood by friends in relation to their pain versus feeling disliked. Overall, they remarked that non-friend peers and others in their communities asked questions and made comments that made them feel stigmatized for having pain.

Peer support has been conceptualized as providing informational, emotional, and appraisal functions and identified as improving health outcomes through numerous actions including reinforcing help-seeking behaviors, encouraging effective coping, promoting social comparisons, and aiding self esteem (18). Half of the participants felt that peers who had pain would provide a major source of support. Those not in favour of this cited the idiosyncratic nature of pain. Lazarus (6) asserts that individuals tend not to seek social support if their self-esteem is at stake. Recent research suggests that chronic pain in adults has a negative impact on one's self and identity which is made worse in the public arena (19). It would be important to know if adolescents not interested in peer support appraised the sharing of their pain as somehow shameful.

Regardless of the positive impact of peer support on various health conditions it remains unclear what form of peer support adolescents with chronic pain would benefit from. We know little about the actual peer relationships of adolescents with chronic pain and even less about what needs would be met through peer support, or, the best method for delivering peer support to these adolescents. There is evidence emerging within adolescent populations that suggests some negative effects of peer support exchanges (20-22). More research is needed before peer support becomes a mainstay in adolescent chronic pain care.

The thought of transition to adult care was overwhelming. They were unsure what skills they needed, were skeptical about adult health care professionals, and asserted they were not ready to transition but felt strongly that they should be involved in the decision of when to transition. Similar to adolescents with other chronic illnesses, chronological age was not seen as the best determinant of readiness; as self-management and advocacy skills are essential for adolescents, regardless of their chronic illness, to navigating the adult care system (23,24). It has also been suggested that some adolescents, by the very nature of their illness, may not receive the same level of expertise by adult health care professionals, such as those living with cystic fibrosis (23). This is pertinent for adolescents with chronic pain as recognition of pain as a disease is fairly recent. Thus, health professionals working in adult chronic pain clinics have not had the opportunity to work with adolescent patients and be aware of their unique needs. Trusting a new adult health care team was concerning, as they had encountered disbelief from health professionals in the past.

Although living with pain present challenges, the adolescents in this study found positive management strategies. Evidence supports the effectiveness of various cognitive behavioral techniques such as guided imagery and relaxation (25,26) but distraction was the primary pain coping strategy and it was adaptable to most situations. Given that coping is an individual process, which changes over time and context, the usefulness of distraction is not surprising.

Even though pacing is regarded as an important strategy for managing chronic pain (27) only one participate found this to be true. The rest stated that they no longer paced activity, as it was not beneficial. These participants approached activity by "packing it in". Pacing may remind them of how they are different from their peers and thus rejected. Recent literature suggests that a formal approach to pacing may be used by some individuals to avoid activity by focusing on rest or shirking pain producing activities, while a functional approach to pacing, which focuses on pacing as a way to reduce pain's influence, may improve functioning (28). How important pacing is remains a matter for discussion, as Nielson et al (29) found that pacing only contributed to 2-4% of the explained variance in functioning of a 110 adults with fibromyalgia after controlling for sex, gender, pain severity, and scores on the Chronic Pain Coping Inventory. It may be that 'packing it' is the adolescents' perception of functional pacing. The one participant who found pacing helpful described purposefully missing out on activities and thus may be using pacing as a reason to avoid activities. It remains unknown how, or to what degree, pacing improves functioning in adolescents with chronic pain.

Since we only gathered data during one session it may be that additionally needs would have been uncovered in subsequent discussions. The goal of qualitative research is not to reach generalizable conclusions; a quantitative study to determine if other adolescents with chronic pain have similar needs is warranted.

Conclusions

Youth attending a tertiary care pain clinic had multiple needs. They struggled to be normal while dealing with their pain. They identified needing help with school and communicating with friends and others about their pain. Friends were important but friendships were negatively impacted by the adolescents' chronic pain. Half the participants viewed support from another peer with chronic pain as positive. Distraction was the favored strategy for coping; pacing was least valued. Transition to adult care evoked several concerns including timing of transition and the needed skills to engage in adult health systems. It would be important for health care professionals to be aware of these self-identified needs in order improve outcomes for adolescents with chronic pain.

Acknowledgments

This research has been funded by a Rising Researcher Support Award from the Child Health Clinician Scientist Program to Paula Forgeron and her PhD studies are support by a Canadian Institutes of Health Research—Doctoral Research Fellowship.

References

[1] Sällfors C, Fasth A, Hallberg LR. Oscillating between hope and despair—a qualitative study. Child Care Health Dev 2002;28:495-505.
[2] Carter B, Lambrenos K, Thursfield J. A pain workshop: An approach to eliciting the views of young people with chronic pain. J Clin Nurs 2002;11:753-62.
[3] Perquin CW, Hazebroek-Kampschreur AA, Hunfeld JA, Bohnen AM, van Suijlekom-Smit LW, Passchier J, van der Wouden JC. Pain in children and adolescents: A common experience. Pain 2000;87: 51-8.
[4] Goodman JE, McGrath PJ. The epidemiology of pain in children and adolescents: A review. Pain 1991;46:247-64.
[5] Bursch B. Pain in infants, children, and adolescents SIG: Policy statement on peditaric chronic pain. APS Bulletin,10, retrieved October 10, 2007 http://www.ampainsoc.org/pub/bulletin/may00/sig1.
[6] Lazarus RS. Coping with the stress of illness. In: Kaplun A, ed. Health promotion and chronic illness. Geneva: WHO, 1992.
[7] Sandelowski M. Whatever happened to qualitative description? Res Nurs Health 2000;23:334-40.
[8] Merriam SB. Qualitative research and case study application in education. San Francisco: Jossey-Bass, 1998.
[9] Morgan DL. Focus groups. Ann Rev Sociol 1996;22:129-52.
[10] Morgan DL. Focus groups. In: Hesse-Biber SN, Leavy P, eds. Approaches to qualitative research: A reader on theory and practice. New York: Oxford Univ Press, 2004:263-85.
[11] Holloway I, Wheeler S. Qualitative research in nursing, 2nd ed. Oxford: Blackwell, 2002.
[12] Lincoln Y, Guba E. Naturalistic inquiry. London: Sage, 1985.
[13] Christensen PH. Childhood and the cultural constitutions of vulnerable bodies. In: Prout A, ed. The body, childhood and society. Basingstoke, UK: MacMillan, 2000:38-59.
[14] James A. Embodied being(s): Understanding the self and the body in childhood. In: Prout A, ed. The body, childhood and society. Basingstoke, UK: MacMillan, 2000:19-37).
[15] Guell C. Painful childhood: children living with juvenile arthritis. Qual Health Res 2007;17:884-92.
[16] Greco LA, Kari E, Freeman MS, Dufton L. Overt and relational victimization among children with frequent abdominal pain: Links to social skills, academic functioning, and health service use. J Pediatr Psychol 2007;32:319-29.
[17] Kashikar-Zuck S, Lynch A, Graham B, Swain N, Mullen SA. Social functioning and peer relationships of adolescents with juvenile fibromyalgia syndrome. Arthritis Rheum 2007;57:474-80.
[18] Dennis C. Peer support within a health care context: a concept analysis. Int J Nurs Stud 2003;40:321-32.
[19] Smith J, Osborn M. Pain as an assault on the self: An interpretative phenomenological analysis of the psychological impact of chronic benign low back pain. Psychol Health 2007;22(5):517-34.
[20] Rose AJ, Carlson W, Waller EM. Prospective associations of co-rumination with friendship and emotional adjustment: Considering the socioemotional trade-offs of co-rumination. Dev Psychol 2007;43:1019-31.
[21] Rose AJ. Co-rumination in the friendships of girls and boys. Child Dev 2002;73:1830-43.

[22] Gramic I, Dishion TJ. Deviant talk in adolescent friendships: A step toward measuring a pathogenic attractor process. Soc Dev 2003;12, 314-34.
[23] Reiss JG, Gibson RW, Walker L. Health care transition: Youth, family, and provider perspectives. Pediatrics 2005;15:112-20.
[24] McDonagh JE. Transition of care from paediatric to adult rheumatology. Arch Dis Child 2007;92:802-7.
[25] McGrath PJ, Humphreys P, Keene D, Goodman JT, Lascelles MA, Cunningham SJ. The efficacy and efficiency of a self-administered treatment for adolescent migraine. Pain 1992;49;321-4.
[26] Hicks CL, von Baeyer C, McGrath PJ. Online psychological treatment for pediatric recurrent pain: A randomized evaluation. J Pediatr Psychol 2006;31:724-36.
[27] Hanson RW, Gerber KE. Coping with chronic pain: a guide to self-management. New York: Guilford, 1990.
[28] McCracken LM, Samuel VM. The role of avoidance, pacing, and other activity patterns in chronic pain. Pain 2007;130:119-25.
[29] Nielson WR, Jensen MP, Hill ML. An activity pacing scale for the chornic pain coping inventory: development in a sample of patients with fibromyalgia syndrome. Pain 2001;89:111-5.

VI. Sickle cell disease

In: Children and Pain
Editors: P. Schofield and J. Merrick ISBN 978-1-60876-020-6

Chapter 9

Clinical trials in children and adolescents with pain and sickle cell disease

Melissa J Frei-Jones, MD[*1,2] *and Michael R DeBaun, MD MPH*[2,3]
[1]Department of Pediatrics,
Washington University School of Medicine,
St Louis, Missouri
[2]Hematology-Oncology, Department of Pediatrics,
University of Texas Health Science Center, San Antonio, Texas
[3]Department of Genetics, Washington University School of Medicine,
St Louis, Missouri, United States of America

Abstract

The number of clinical trials in Sickle Cell Disease (SCD) has increased over the past 20 years. New knowledge and a better understanding of the pathophysiology of SCD has made a tremendous impact on survival and long-term morbidity.

Despite improvements, SCD-pain remains the most common and debilitating morbidity experienced by individuals with SCD regardless of genotype. We systematically reviewed all prospective clinical trials for the treatment of pain among children and adolescents with SCD. For comparison, a search was also performed to identify all prospective pain clinical trials of morphine for the treatment of post-operative pain in children and adolescents without SCD.

* Correspondence: Assistant Professor Melissa Frei-Jones, MD, Msci, Hematology-Oncology, Department of Pediatrics, University of Texas Health Science Center, 333 N. Santa Rosa, RM B8208, San Antonio, TX 78207 United States. E-mail: FreiJones@uthscsa.edu

Introduction

The number of clinical trials in Sickle Cell Disease (SCD) has increased over the past 20 years. New knowledge and a better understanding of the pathophysiology of SCD has made a tremendous impact on survival and long-term morbidity. Despite improvements, SCD-pain remains the most common and debilitating morbidity experienced by individuals with SCD regardless of genotype. SCD pain, with or without utilization of care, is more prevalent than previously acknowledge. In a cohort study of 232 adults with SCD followed for six months, pain occurred in 50% of reported days (1). Natural history studies have been useful, increasing our understanding when describing the incidence and severity of pain. However, the lack of a uniform definition of pain greatly limits our ability to generalize the results. More importantly, the lack of uniform pain definitions limits comparability of clinical trials.

To better define the use of pain as a primary outcome measure in clinical trials in children with SCD, we systematically reviewed all prospective clinical trials for the treatment of pain among children and adolescents with SCD. For comparison, a search was also performed to identify all prospective pain clinical trials of morphine for the treatment of post-operative pain in children and adolescents without SCD.

Study identification

Searches were conducted on the following computerized bibliographic databases (Figure I): Medline Database (January 1980-January 2008) using Ovid (http://gateway.ovid.com/) and PubMed (http://www.ncbi.nlm.nih.gov/sites/entrez/), Embase (http://www.embase.com/; January 1980-January 2008), Web of Science (http://www.embase.com/;January 1988-January 2008) and the Cochran Clinical Trials Registry (http://www3.interscience.wiley.com/cgi-bin/mrwhome/106568753/HOME; as of January 2008). The time period of 1980-2008 was chosen due to the paucity of randomized clinical trials in children prior to 1980.

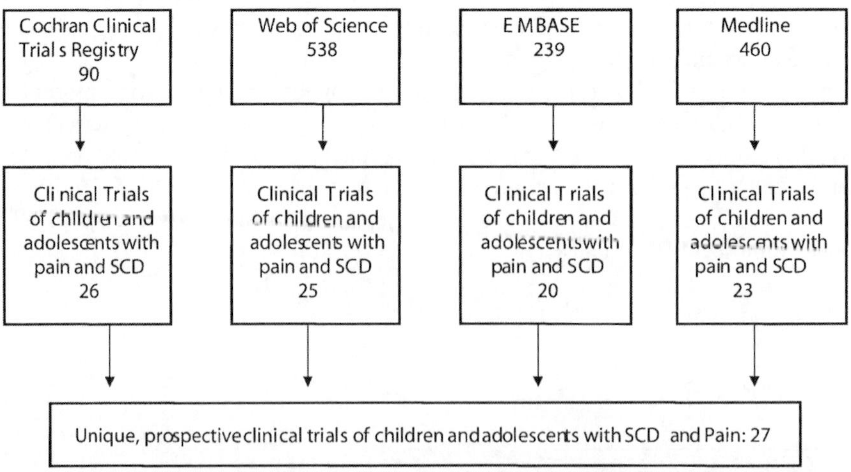

Figure 1. Literature Search Schema.

SCD pain in children

The search terms used for the primary literature search were: 1) Sickle cell disease or sickle cell anemia, 2) pain or vaso-occlusive pain or vaso-occlusive episode or vaso-occlusive crisis and 3) clinical trial. In addition, the bibliographies of all review articles and all selected articles were examined. Study titles and abstracts were evaluated and all studies meeting the following criteria were included: prospective clinical trials including children (infants to 18 years) and/or adults with any form of Sickle Cell Disease. Case reports, retrospective studies, descriptive cohort studies, and review articles were not included.

The first and second search terms produced 90 clinical trials from The Cochran Clinical Trials Registry; 538 references from the Web of Science; 239 references from EMBASE; and 460 references from Medline. After excluding all case reports, review articles, retrospective studies and choosing only clinical trials including adolescents and children with SCD, 26 references met criteria from the The Cochran Clinical Trials Registry; 25 from the Web of Science; 20 from EMBASE; and 23 from Medline. Ultimately, 27 unique studies were identified (see table 1) (2-28). Given that retrospective, observational studies and case-reports did not meet criteria for inclusion in this review, a separate table describing these studies were included (see table 2) (29-38) to demonstrate the paucity of prospective studies.

Post-operative pain in children

Search terms used for the secondary literature search were: 1) pain, 2) morphine sulfate, 3) child and 4) clinical trial. The bibliographies of all review articles and selected articles were examined; all studies meeting the following criteria were included: prospective clinical trials in children (infants to 18 years) who received intravenous morphine sulfate for the treatment of post-operative pain. Trials involving the administration of epidural, intramuscular or caudal morphine sulfate were not included because these methodologies are not currently used to treat SCD Pain. Literature searches produced 22 references from the Cochrane Clinical Trials registry; 60 references from PubMed Central; 51 references from EMBASE; 5 references from Web of Science and 48 references from Ovid Medline. Twenty-two unique trials were identified from the literature searches that met all inclusion criteria (39-60).

Clinical trials in pain medications for symptomatic treatment

Opioid analgesics

Morphine

The most common approach to the treatment of moderate to severe pain, whether SCD-related or due to some other cause, is the administration of an opioid analgesic for symptomatic relief. In clinical practice, the opioid most frequently chosen to treat SCD-pain is morphine.

Table 1. Prospective Clinical Trials in Children and Adolescents with Pain and SCD

Citation	N	Age (yrs)	Study Design	Treatment	Pain Definition	Pain Scores	Outcomes	Adverse Events
Christensen ML, et al., 1996.(2)	10	9-16	Single arm	Transdermal Fentanyl	Acute, requiring hospital admission and opioid administration	-clinical and verbal pain assessment	-No difference in morphine use. -Delay in reaching therapeutic concentration.	-Prolonged delay in reaching therapeutic concentrations.
Jacobson SJ, et al., 1997. (3)	56	5-17	RCT Double-blind, Placebo-controlled	Oral vs IV Morphine	Acute pain in extremities, back, abdomen and chest due to SCD.	-Self-report and behavioral -CHEOPS -faces scale -Oucher African-American Scale	-No difference in supplemental analgesics. -No difference in pain scores.	- none reported
Melzer-Lange MD, et al., 2004 (4)	69	10-18	Pilot study, Randomized by Treating Physician	Morphine PCA started early in the ED or later in the Inpatient Unit	VOC	-No pain assessment	-Protocol successful in decreasing time to PCA start. -Patients preferred PCA started in ED.	- none reported
Robieux IC, et al., 1992. (5)	66	3-18	For PCA - "Before-After" Design For Oxygen - RCT Double-blind, Placebo-controlled	Intermittent IV vs PCA Morphine Oxygen vs Placebo in patients receiving PCA only	Hospitalized for acute SCD pain	-Behavioral observational scale	- No difference in equivalent morphine dose. -Shorter LOS for patients receiving PCA -No difference between oxygen and placebo	-none reported
Hardwick WE Jr, et al., 1999. (6).	29	5-18	RCT, Double-blind, Placebo-controlled	Ketorolac + Morphine vs Placebo + Morphine	Pain crisis	-Self-report -10-cm VAS	-No difference in VAS scores. -No difference in morphine use. -No difference in LOS and ED return.	- none reported
Beiter JL Jr, et al., 2001. (7)	51	6-18	Single-arm	Ketorolac	Vaso-occlusive pain	-Self-report -Nine FACES pain scale -100-mm VAS	-Patients with mild to mod pain (VAS<70-mm) can be treated with ketorolac alone. -Patients with VAS>70-mm required opioid analgesia and admission.	- none reported

Citation	N	Age (yrs)	Study Design	Treatment	Pain Definition	Pain Scores	Outcomes	Adverse Events
Perlin E, et al., 1994. (8)	21	≥ 15	RCT Placebo-controlled	Ketorolac vs Meperidine	Acute VOC	-Self-report -0 to 3 verbal categorical scale -100-mm VAS	-Continuous ketorolac was superior to as needed IM meperidine in pain relief -Fewer doses of meperidine were used by patients receiving ketorolac	- GI upset.
Grisham JE, et al., 1996. (9)	20	11-19	Randomized, Crossover	Ketorolac vs Meperidine	Acute pain episode	-Self-report -80-mm VAS	-Lower pain scores at 30 min, but difference did not persist	-none reported
de Franceschi L, et al., 2004. (10)	7	16-30	Pilot Study, Prospective Case Series	Ketorolac, Tramadol and Transfusion	VOC	-Self-report -0 to 10 VAS	-Shorter hospital LOS than historical controls.	- none reported
Eke FU, et al., 2000. (11)	58	3-14	RCT Parallel Design	Piroxicam vs Soluble Acetylsalicylic Acid	Osteoarticular painful attack	-Self-report -5-point verbal scale	-piroxicam was superior to aspirin	-GI discomfort with aspirin
Greenberg J, et al., 1993. (12)	49	2-17	Crossover Double-blind Placebo-controlled	Aspirin vs Placebo	Pain crisis	-No self-report -Calculated pain score	- no difference between aspirin and placebo	- none reported.
Zago MA, et al., 1984. (13)	29	4-31	RCT Placebo-controlled	Aspirin vs Placebo	Pain crisis	-No pain assessment	-no difference between aspirin and placebo	-none reported.
Griffin TC, et al., 1994. (14).	36	2-19	RCT Double-blind Placebo-controlled	IV Methyl-prednisolone	Acute pain that remained severe after home treatment.	-No pain assessment	-shorter duration of inpatient analgesia.	-higher readmission rate

Table 1. (Continued)

Citation	N	Age (yrs)	Study Design	Treatment	Pain Definition	Pain Scores	Outcomes	Adverse Events
Weiner DL, et al., 2003. (15)	20	10-21	RCT Double-blind, Placebo-controlled	Inhaled Nitric Oxide	Uncomplicated, severe acute VOC with a score of ≥ 6-cm on a 10-cm VAS scale.	-Self-report -10-cm VAS	- Pain scores not statistically different between groups. - Less IV opioids in the INO - No difference in LOS	-none reported
Brousseau DC, et al., 2004. (16)	19	4-18	Single-arm, Historical Controls	IV Magnesium	Sickle cell pain crisis	-No pain assessment	-shorter LOS and quantity of opioids used with magnesium.	-1 patient readmitted -1 episode hypotension
Zipursky A, et al., 1992. (17).	25	3-18	RCT	Oxygen vs Room air	Acute, painful VOC requiring admission	-McGrath Behavioral Pain Scale	- fewer RSCs - no change in clinical course of pain	- none reported.
Miller ST, et al., 2001.(18)	130	2-16	RCT	Transfusion vs standard care	Pain in the extremities, back, abdomen, chest or head for which no other explanation could be found lasting at least 2 hours and requiring a medical visit.	-No pain assessment	- fewer pain episodes when analyzed by treatment received. -intent to treat analysis was not significant.	- none reported
Bouchaïr N, et al., 2000. (19)	7	4-24	Prospective Cohort, Before-and-After; Hgb > 9.5 gm/dL	Phlebotomy	More than 3 pain crises in the year before.	-No pain assessment	- fewer days in hospital	- none reported - only relevant for patients with high hgb levels.
Wang WC, et al., 1988. (20)	22	12-27	RCT Double-blind Placebo-controlled	TENS	Stratification by severity of crisis: Grade I or mild pain- pain score 1-4, relief with oral meds and no hospitalization; Grade II or moderate pain - pain score 5-7, relief with oral meds and no hospitalization; Grade III or severe pain - pain score 8-10, relief after dose of parenteral opioids, and no hospitalization Grade IV or severe pain - with pain score 8-10, little or no relief from parenteral opioids and hospitalized	-Self-report -0 to 10 VAS	- no difference in pain scores - no difference in analgesic use	- none reported

Citation	N	Age (yrs)	Study Design	Treatment	Pain Definition	Pain Scores	Outcomes	Adverse Events
Gil KM, et al., 2001. (21)	46	8-17	RCT	Coping Skills	Defined by patient in diary.	-Self-report -0-10 numerical scale	-Less healthcare contact when coping skills used -Less school absence when coping skills used.	- none reported.
Wambebe C, et al., 2001. (22)	84	10-29	Crossover Double-blind Placebo-controlled	Niprisan	Acute painful event requiring treatment at a healthcare facility or at home with parenteral opioids, equianalgesic doses of oral opioids, parenteral NSAIDs, or equianalgesic doses of oral NSAIDs	-No pain assessment	- Fewer pain episodes when taking study drug. - Less missed days of work.	- headache - rash
Jayabose S, et al., 1996. (23)	15	4-18	Open-label, Single-arm Pilot Study	Hydroxyurea	SCD pain was defined as any painful episode involving the extremities, abdomen, back or chest, including ACS that resulted in hospitalization.	-No pain assessment	-Significant decrease in number of pain episodes.	- asymptomatic neutropenia -hair loss -nausea -elevated hemoglobin
Karimi M, et al., 2006. (24)	17	5-34	Single-blind, Placebo-controlled Crossover	Cromolyn Sodium Nasal Spray and Hydroxyurea	VOC	-Self-report -Wong-Baker FACES Scale	-No difference between cromolyn sodium and placebo in pain scores.	-no toxicities reported from cromolyn
Alvim RC, et al., 2005. (25)	73	5-20	Crossover Double-blind Placebo-controlled	Piracetam	VOC in the limbs, vertebral spine, thorax or abdomen, of variable intensity and duration, without other identifiable cause, with or without medical assistance, preferably recognized by patients and relatives as the characteristic pain caused by the disease	-Self-report -VAS	- No difference between piracetam and placebo	-none reported

Table 1. (Continued)

Citation	N	Age (yrs)	Study Design	Treatment	Pain Definition	Pain Scores	Outcomes	Adverse Events
Adams-Graves P, et al., 1997. (26)	50	15-55	Randomized, Double-blind, Placebo-controlled Pilot Study	PP188	Moderate or severe pain, typical of usual painful event, lasting at least 4 hours but not more than 18 hours requiring admission for parenteral analgesics	-Self-report -5-point 0-3 verbal scale	-Shorter LOS -Less analgesics needed. -Lower pain intensity scores.	-Headache, nausea, abdominal pain and constipation. -one serious event: elevated creatinine after study drug delivery in patient with underlying renal insufficiency
Orringer EP, et al., 2001. (27)	255, 73 child	12-30	RCT Double-blind, Placebo-controlled	PP188	Sudden onset of acute pain in ≥ 1 sites typical of vaso-occlusive crisis requiring parenteral analgesics	-Self-report -100-mm VAS	-Duration of pain 21 hour shorter in subset of children receiving PP188.	-No renal complications. -One death due to pulmonary fat embolism in one pt received PP188
Manrique RV., 1987. (28)	60	7-34	RCT Double-blind, Placebo-controlled	Pento-xifylline	Type A - patients who experience permanent pain in muscles, bones, joints or mixed without fever or other organ involvement. Type B - patients with intermittent pain in muscles, bones, joints or mixed without fever or other organ involvement; Type C - painful crises in muscles, bones and joints with fever, organ involvement and pronounced hemolysis	-Self-report - 4-point verbal pain scale	-Shorter duration of pain -Lower pain scores	-GI upset and shivering not different between study drug and placebo.

LOS = Length of Stay; INO = Inhaled Nitrous Oxide; VAS = Visual Analog Scale; PCA = Patient Controlled Analgesia; IV = Intravenous; VOC = Vaso-Occlusive Crisis; RSC = Reversible Sickled Cells; RCT = Randomized Controlled Trial; Hydroxyurea = HU; Poloxamer 188 = PP188; Transcutaneous Electrical Nerve Stimulator = TENS; Children of Eastern Ontario Pain Scale = CHEOPS.

Table 2. Retrospective Clinical Trials and Case Reports in Children and Adolescents with Pain and SCD

Citation	N	Age (yrs)	Study Design	Treatment	Pain Defn	Outcomes/Results	Risks
Buchanan ID, et al., 2005.(29)	175	5-19	Retrospective chart review	IV Nalbuphine vs IV Morphine	VOC, ICD-9 Codes 282.60 and 282.62	-ACS less frequent in pts receiving Nalbuphine (26 vs 11, $p<.01$) -Shorter LOS (3 vs 4 days with Nalbuphine.)	-No additional reported.
Carbajal R , et al., 1996.(30)	2	11	Case Report	Inhaled Nitrous Oxide for pain not relieved by continuous morphine.	VOC	-15-20 minutes of 50% inhaled nitrous oxide provided complete and sustained pain relief (3 hrs).	-No desaturations.
Holbrook CT, et al., 1990. (31)	20	≤18	Retrospective	PCA versus intermittent scheduled opioids	VOC	-More rapid pain relief with PCA. -Patients and families preferred PCA. -Total IV opioid dose higher in PCA group. -No difference in LOS.	-None reported.
Huehns ER, et al., 1981.(32)	11	5-32	Retrospective	Fresh Frozen Plasma	Painful VOC	-Shorter LOS. -Lower opioid use. -Improved patient-reported pain relief.	-Did not prevent development of ACS.
Kopecky EA, et al., 2004.(33)	50	5-17	Post-hoc analysis of RCT trial	Oral vs IV morphine	VOC - severe debilitating pain.	-More ACS developed in pts receiving oral morphine (57% vs 17%)	-No additional reported.
Schechter NL, et al., 1988.(34)	3	11-17	Case Report	PCA	VOC	-Adolescents with SCD could be taught to use a PCA successfully.	-None reported.
Styles LA, et al., 1994. (35)	17	4-16	Retrospective Before-and-after	Chronic Transfusion	Pain requiring hospitalization and opioids without a non-SCD cause.	-Significant decrease in number of painful events and hospitalizations during transfusion therapy.	- None reported.

Table 2. (Continued)

Trentadue NO, et al., 1998.(36)	26	Child	Retrospective chart review	Comparing two types of PCA	Sickle Cell pain crisis	-Pts receiving a low basal infusion and high PCA dose used less morphine and had shorter LOS than pts receiving high basal infusion with low PCA dose.	-None reported.
Woods GM, et al., 1990.(37)	16	≤18	Retrospective review	IM meperidine vs IM nalbuphine	Painful episodes	-Nalbuphine as effective as IM meperidine.	-None reported.
Yaster M, et al., 1994.(38)	9	3-16	Retrospective, cohort	Epidural analgesia with local anesthetic alone or with fentanyl	VOC	-Rapid decrease in pain (within 15 min) in 8 of 9 patients. -Improved PaO2 with epidural use.	-One catheter dislodged. -One post-dural puncture headache.

LOS = Length of Stay; INO = Inhaled Nitrous Oxide; VAS = Visual Analog Scale; PCA = Patient Controlled Analgesia; IV = Intravenous; IM = Intramuscular; VOC = Vaso-Occlusive Crisis; RSC = Reversible Sickled Cells; RCT = Randomized Controlled Trial; Hydroxyurea = HU; Poloxamer 188 = PP188; Transcutaneous Electrical Nerve Stimulator = TENS; Children of Eastern Ontario Pain Scale = CHEOPS.

The literature review identified three trials evaluating method of morphine delivery and one trial comparing morphine to ketorolac. These four trials will be discussed in subsequent sections. No trials comparing morphine to an alternative opioid were identified as part of a prospective clinical trial among children with SCD. Several retrospective studies were identified [29-31, 33-34, 36]; however, these studies were not included.

Fentanyl

Fentanyl use, in general, has increased due to its shorter half-life, allowing for more rapid titration, and more favorable side effect profile. A single study evaluating the use of fentanyl in children with SCD was identified. Christensen, et al. performed a single-arm, unblinded, prospective study evaluating the efficacy of transdermal fentanyl and correlation with serum fentanyl levels[2]. Efficacy of pain relief was determined using clinical and verbal pain assessments as well as amount of supplemental patient controlled analgesia (PCA) doses of morphine. Either a 25 mcg/hr or a 50 mcg/hr transdermal patch was placed on the chest wall depending upon the amount of morphine received in the previous 24 hours. Pain was assessed using a categorical pain scale (0 to 9).

A Sickle Cell pain crisis (SCPC) was defined as an acute condition requiring opioid administration in the hospital. The authors report no difference in pain scores between the study intervals. The amount of supplemental morphine decreased from 0.83 mg/kg/day to 0.38 mg/kg/day during the first 24 hours, with total opioid use increasing to 1.98 mg/kg/day when morphine equivalents of fentanyl were included.

Of note, half of the patients studied did not reach the minimum effective serum fentanyl concentrations until 24-hrs after transdermal patch placement. No follow-up studies or other trials of intravenous fentanyl were located in the literature review.

Meperidine

An alternative opioid analgesic, meperidine has more frequently been the subject of clinical trials in adults, but due to significant adverse effects including neurotoxicity and seizures, is less often used in the treatment of pediatric SCD-pain. Although meperidine is clinically popular, no clinical trials comparing the efficacy of meperidine with morphine or any other opioid analgesic in children was found in the literature review. Two trials comparing meperidine and ketorolac were identified and will be discussed in a subsequent section.

Hydromorphone

Hydromorphone, a more potent opioid analgesic, is often used in adolescents and adults who experience inadequate relief with morphine. No clinical trials of hydromorphone for the treatment of SCD-pain in children were identified in this review.

Nalbuphine

Nalbuphine, one of a number of mixed opioid agonist/antagonists, has become standard therapy for SCD-pain in some medical centers. However, only one retrospective analysis of the efficacy of nalbuphine in treating sickle cell pain in children was published in 1990 (37). No follow-up prospective or randomized trials were found in the literature review.

Oral versus intravenous opioids

Opioid analgesics may be administered locally or systemically, by topical, oral, intra-nasal, rectal, intramuscular, intravenous or epidural route. In the United States, the approach to SCD-pain in children requiring hospital admission is to administer parenteral opioids. Stronger oral opioids are now available and include the morphine derivatives oxycodone, oxycontin, morphine sulfate-immediate release and morphine sulfate-sustained release.

A single trial was identified comparing oral and intravenous (IV) opioid administration. Jacobson, et al. published a prospective, double-blind, placebo-controlled, randomized trial comparing IV and oral morphine in children hospitalized with SCD-pain (3). The study objective was to compare the efficacy of extended-release oral morphine to morphine administered by continuous infusion. SCD-pain was defined as pain in the extremities, back, abdomen and chest that could not be explained except by SCD. Pain was assessed using a faces pain scale, the Oucher African-American pain scale, the children of Eastern Ontario pain scale (CHEOPS), and a five-point clinical pain assessment. The primary measure of efficacy was the five-point clinical pain score. The authors reported no difference in rate of rescue analgesia or in pain scores reported using the Oucher, CHEOPS or five-point clinical pain scale. The studied concluded oral opioids were as effective as IV opioids in the management of pediatric SCD-pain and may allow for improved outpatient pain management. However, in this study, regular dose escalation was done every 12-hrs by physicians for both patients receiving oral and IV morphine and doses were delivered around-the-clock. The authors reported wide variability in the amount of oral morphine needed to produce pain relief. It is unlikely that such aggressive dose escalation could be easily replicated within the home.

Patient controlled analgesia

After hospital admission for treatment of SCD-pain, IV analgesics may be delivered by intermittent dosing based on the half life of the opioid or by using patient controlled analgesia (PCA) with a continuous basal infusion and patient-administered bolus doses. In example, for morphine administration, the clinician has two choices: to give IV morphine every two or three hours or give a morphine continuous infusion with PCA administration. Moderate to severe vaso-occlusive pain in children with SCD requiring admission to the hospital should almost never be treated with as needed (prn) intravenous opioids. The administration of prn opioids is rarely successful except when another factor, such as fever, and not the pain episode itself necessitated admission. Further, in many hospitals, the nursing guidelines allow for prn medication to be given within an hour of patient request. Such a long interval between the request for pain medication by the patient and/or caregiver and the delivery of the medication, coupled with the additional time required for the onset of pain relief after administration, may result in at least a 1.5 hour interval between the request for pain medication and pain relief.

Two prospective clinical trials evaluating the use of PCA in children with SCD-pain were identified. The first trial evaluated the ability of an ED protocol to shorten time to PCA initiation, patient preference and length of stay[4]. Patients were randomized by treating physician to either ED or inpatient PCA initiation. Pain was defined as moderate to severe vaso-occlusive pain requiring hospitalization and pain scores were not assessed. Among patients who received both forms of PCA, 92% (23 of 25) preferred PCA initiation in the ED rather than on the hospital floor. Length of stay was the same between groups. For patients who started their PCA after admission to the floor, the average time between last dose of analgesia in the ED and PCA initiation was 211 +/- 17 minutes. Such a long time interval between leaving the ED and starting the PCA on the floor is an opportunity for improvement in medical care and patient/family satisfaction.

The second clinical trial sought to compare the efficacy of intermittent-dose IV opioids versus continuous infusion morphine using a prospective, before-and-after study design as well as determine the pharmacokinetics and pharmacodynamics of continuous IV morphine (5). Secondarily, they sought to determine if 50% face mask oxygen versus placebo would decrease the duration of pain in patients receiving continuous IV morphine which will be discussed in a later section. SCD pain was defined as a severe vaso-occlusive crisis (VOC). Pain was assessed using the behavioral observation scale (BPS). Patients received three possible types of intermittent IV opioids, codeine, meperidine or morphine, but all patients assigned to continuous infusion received morphine. No difference in morphine equivalent dose was found between the two groups. The duration of severe pain was shorter in patients receiving continuous IV morphine than intermittent dose, suggesting that continuous infusion was superior to intermittent dosing.

Home management

The majority of SCD-pain experienced by children and adolescents does not require hospitalization; rather it is managed at home by the patients and their caregivers [61]. No prospective clinical trials regarding the home management of SCD-pain in children or adolescents were identified.

Non-steroidal anti-inflammatory agents

Ibuprofen

Severe pain is not only treated with opioid analgesics but frequently is accompanied by adjuvant analgesics such as non-steroidal anti-inflammatory (NSAIDs) medications. Although ibuprofen is the most commonly used oral NSAID, no published studies in children or adolescents with SCD and pain exist. The cyclo-oxygenase 2 (COX-2) inhibitor, rofecoxib was evaluated in a pharmacokinetic study[62] but was removed from the market shortly after publication. No other COX-2 inhibitors have been investigated.

Ketorolac

Ketorolac is the only parenteral NSAID studied in children and adolescents with SCD and pain; its use is often controversial. The literature revealed two studies using ketorolac as upfront analgesic therapy in the ED, two studies comparing the efficacy of ketorolac with meperidine and one pilot study using ketorolac, tramadol and transfusion therapy.

Ketorolac in the ED

The first ED study randomized patients, ages 5-17, in a double-blind fashion to receive IV ketorolac versus placebo plus adjuvant morphine. The authors hypothesized that a single dose of ketorolac would decrease the amount of adjuvant morphine needed, hospitalization rate and ED return rate when compared to morphine alone (6). SCD-pain was defined as a pain crisis. Pain was assessed using a 10-cm linear visual analog scale (VAS). The authors found no significant difference in VAS scores, additional morphine use, or hospitalization rate. Hospital readmission after initial inpatient treatment was not evaluated. No significant adverse effects were reported. Although the ED return rate was not statistically different between groups, more patients who received ketorolac returned to the ED after initial discharge than those given placebo (23%, 3/11 vs 0%, 0/9). This trend suggests one-dose of ketorolac may be helpful to temporarily improve pain allowing for ED discharge but is insufficient to abort a pain episode, resulting in rebound pain.

The second trial evaluated the use of ketorolac, rather than an opioid, as initial therapy for SCD-pain upon presentation to the ED in a single arm, non-blinded study (7). Consecutive patients, ages 6-18, received 0.5-1 mg/kg IV ketorolac; no placebo or control group was included. SCD-pain was defined as vaso-occlusive pain secondary to a sickle hemoglobinopathy. Pain was assessed using a 100-mm VAS and a Nine Faces Pain Scale (NFPS). Patients with an initial VAS of 50-60 were able to be discharged after one dose. Patients with an initial VAS of 70-80 required additional analgesics and were ultimately admitted. For patients with milder pain, 13% (4/32) returned to the ED within 48 hours for additional analgesics. The authors concluded patients with mild pain could be treated successfully with ketorolac rather than an opioid but those with moderate to severe pain required opioid-based therapy.

Based on these two studies, ketorolac does not appear to have any advantage in the treatment of moderate to severe SCD-pain. Ketorolac has not been shown to decrease pain scores, hospitalization rate or adjuvant morphine use. Although some benefit may be seen in patients with milder pain, careful attention should be paid to the number of patients who return after initial treatment (and compared to the reported ED return within 72 hours for patients treated with opioids-alone of 11% (11/101) (63).

Ketorolac and meperidine

In the first trial, Perlin et al (8) randomized adolescents and adults with SCD-pain between continuous IV ketorolac or placebo with supplemental intramuscular (IM) meperidine. SCD pain was defined as moderate to severe pain due to an acute vaso-occlusive crisis. Pain was assessed using a 0 to 3 verbal scale and a 100-mm VAS. The primary efficacy endpoint was amount of additional meperidine needed. Patients receiving continuous IV ketorolac required 33% less meperidine than patients receiving meperidine alone. The generalizability of this trial is limited, because continuous IV ketorolac is not a recommended method of ketorolac administration due to nephrotoxicity and intramuscular opioid injection is considered non-standard care in pediatrics.

In the second trial, a randomized cross-over design, adolescents with SCD-pain received either IV ketorolac or IV meperidine (9). SCD-pain was defined as an acute pain episode. Pain was measured using an 80-mm VAS. The patients who received ketorolac had significantly lower self-report pain scores at 30 minutes than patients receiving meperidine ($p<0.01$) but the difference was not clinically relevant. More patients were discharged home after ketorolac than after meperidine (4 vs 2, $p<0.01$). Meperidine is no longer recommended for the treatment of SCD-pain in children and ketorolac has not been shown to have any advantages to morphine-alone, this study has limited relevance to improving clinical practice for treating SCD related pain.

Ketorolac, tramadol and erythrocytapheresis

The final study including ketorolac described a prospective case series using ketorolac and tramadol coupled with erythrocytapheresis for the treatment of acute SCD-pain in children (10). Primary outcomes were pain relief, length of hospital stay and pain management failure. SCD- pain was defined as an acute VOC and pain was assessed using a 0-10 VAS. Length of stay (LOS) was shorter in the patients receiving erythrocytapheresis than historical controls (6.9 ± 1.5 vs 10.8 ± 0.7 days; $p < 0.05$). The standard treatment received by historical controls was not described and LOS was significantly longer than previously reported in children. This pilot study combined three very different treatment modalities and discerning which treatment provided the most benefit is difficult. Given the poor study design and added cost and inconvenience and risk of erythrocytapheresis, such a study is unlikely to be of practical use among children with sickle cell disease.

Aspirin as analgesic

A single, international trial of aspirin for SCD-pain was identified. Eke, et al. evaluated the use of once-daily piroxicam, an oral NSAID, compared to soluble aspirin in a randomized, parallel-group study (11). SCD-pain was defined as a severe osteoarticular painful attack. Pain and mobility were assessed using five-point scales. Patients receiving piroxicam experienced improved pain control compared to patients who received aspirin. The authors reported combined mean pain scores over 3 days of 1.93 vs 7.73, $p<0.05$. Mean mobility scores were also lower in patients receiving piroxicam on the third hospital day, (0.2 vs 2.2; $p<0.05$). Nausea and abdominal discomfort were more common in the aspirin treated group. These results may not be generalizable to areas where other analgesics are more commonly used for SCD-pain or where aspirin-based therapies are contraindicated due to concerns of Reye Syndrome. Additionally, NSAIDs may result in both gastrointestinal and renal vascular compromise leading to gastric bleeding or renal complications (64,65).

Clinical trials in pain evaluating other medical interventions

A limited number of trials have been conducted with non-analgesic or atypical analgesic medications to decrease the intensity and or duration of SCD-pain episodes. Published clinical trials have investigated the use of glucocorticoids, inhaled nitric oxide, intravenous magnesium therapy, prophylactic oxygen therapy, and transcutaneous nerve stimulation in the treatment of acute SCD-pain.

Table 3. Number Needed to Treat (NNT) and Number Needed to Harm (NNH) in Prospective Clinical Trials to Reduce Frequency of SCD-Pain in Children and Adolescents

Treatment	ARR	NNT	NNH
Chronic Transfusion (18)	Intent to Treat Analysis = 13.9% By Actual Treatment = 25%	7 4	No serious harms reported.
Niprisan (22)	Severe Pain = 37% Hospitalized Pain Episodes = 2%	3 33	No serious harms reported.
Hydroxyurea (23)	Pain Episodes/Patient Year = 12%	8	Asymptomatic Neutropenia = 14

ARR - Absolute Risk Reduction = Event Rate in Control Group - Event Rate in Treatment Group.
NNT - Number Needed to Treat = number of patients who would have to receive therapy to prevent on episode of pain.
NNH - Number Needed to Harm = number of patients who would have to receive therapy for one patient to experience the harmful outcome.

Simple transfusion

The use of simple transfusions during an acute SCD-pain episode in children or adults has not been evaluated prospectively. No evidence exists that a simple blood transfusion will hasten recovery to baseline.

Glucocorticoids

The significant contribution of inflammation to SCD and its associated morbidities has become more apparent. Glucocorticoids are potent, commonly used, anti-inflammatory medications. A single trial evaluating the effect of glucocorticoids in SCD-pain was identified (14). The authors designed a double-blind, placebo-controlled trial of IV methylprednisolone to determine if glucocorticoid administration would shorten length of SCD-pain. Outcome measures included number of morphine doses, need for continuous morphine infusion, duration of IV and oral analgesia and clinical complications. SCD-pain was defined as acute pain that remained severe despite home management. Patient reported pain was not assessed. Age-adjusted duration of inpatient analgesics was less for patients receiving methylprednisolone than placebo (31 vs 62.5 hrs; p = .010). The analysis was repeated after excluding patients who participated more than once or had excessively short visits (< 5hours). The difference between methylprednisolone and placebo persisted (35.8 vs 53.6; p = .012). A higher number of patients who received methylprednisolone were readmitted after discharge than in the placebo group (15%, 4/26 vs 3%, 1/30). The authors concluded the use of methylprednisolone to treat acute SCD-pain may not be advantageous due to the higher than expected readmission rate. A second trial evaluating the use of dexamethasone, an alternative glucocorticoid, for the treatment of acute chest syndrome reported a higher readmission rate within 72 hours after steroid administration of 27% (6/22), mostly for rebound pain (83%, 5/6) (66). Glucocorticoid administration has not been further investigated for the treatment of SCD-pain.

Inhaled Nitric Oxide

Increasing evidence indicates that patients with SCD may have an absolute or relative deficiency in nitric oxide (42). A single trial was identified investigating the use of Inhalational nitric oxide in SCD-pain. Weiner, et al. described the use of inhaled nitric oxide (INO) in a prospective, double-bind trial in older children and adolescents with SCD-pain (15). SCD-pain was defined as an uncomplicated, acute, severe vaso-occlusive crisis with patient-reported pain score of = 6-cm on a 10-cm VAS. Primary outcome measure was change in pain score after 4 hours of INO or placebo therapy. Pain was assessed using a 10-cm undemarcated, horizontal VAS administered by the same investigator. The authors did not clearly define if the investigator was masked to treatment assignment. The study did not find any significant difference in VAS score for patients receiving INO when compared to placebo (2 vs 1.2 cm; p =.37). Patients receiving INO required less IV opioids during the six-hour study period (mean cumulative morphine use, 0.29 vs 0.44 mg/kg, p=0.03) but the difference in hospital LOS was not significant (78 vs 100 hrs, p=0.19). The authors concluded the trial did not succeed in establishing the efficacy or safety of INO in SCD-pain.

Using NO to abate acute painful episodes is an active area of investigation. A search using the terms, Sickle Cell Disease, NO and children on the website, www.clinicaltrials.gov, identified three ongoing or recently completed trials. A phase II, randomized, double-blind, placebo controlled trial evaluating the effectiveness and safety of iNO during acute SCD-pain in patients age 9-22 years has been open since 2005 and scheduled to close September 2008. A second phase II, randomized, double-blind, placebo-controlled trial of iNO during acute SCD-Pain in patients age 10 and older has been opened since 2004 and is scheduled to close June 2008. The third trial employed a different strategy-arginine to increase endogenous NO production rather than iNO. Study design was randomized, double-blind, placebo-controlled with parallel assignment and closed January 2008. Publication of these studies in the near future may change current therapeutic recommendations.

Magnesium

Magnesium, when given intravenously, produces vasodilation and endothelial-dependent release of nitric oxide. A single trial was identified investigating the use of magnesium in SCD-pain (16). Brousseau et al (16) hypothesized IV magnesium would decrease the LOS in children admitted for SCD pain. The study design was non-randomized and patients served as their own controls. Patient-reported pain was not assessed. The authors reported a shorter LOS during the admission where patients received magnesium when compared to their previous admissions for pain (3 vs 5 days; p=0.006). One patient was readmitted within 7 days of discharge and 1 patient developed transient hypotension after magnesium administration that responded to fluid bolus. The authors concluded magnesium warranted further investigation for use in SCD-pain.

Oxygen

The abnormal hemoglobin S in SCD is more unstable in its deoxygenated state when compared to hemoglobin S. Based on the premise that hypoxemia may result in an increase irreversible sickle cells, and ultimately vaso-occlusive pain episode, oxygen may be a reasonable therapeutic intervention. Two studies evaluated the use of oxygen for the treatment of SCD-pain. Both studies were published by the same research team.

The first publication by Robieux et al (5) has been discussed previously as the authors primarily evaluated continuous morphine infusion versus intermittent dose IV opioids to decrease SCD-pain. The patients who received continuous infusion morphine were also randomized to receive 50% supplemental oxygen, regardless of room air oxygen saturations, versus room air. SCD pain was defined as a severe vaso-occlusive crisis (VOC). Pain was assessed using the behavioral observation scale (BPS). They found no difference in duration of severe pain between groups (0.94 vs 0.95 days, p=NS). In general, the use of prophylactic oxygen therapy is not recommended because it masks oxygen desaturation, an early symptom of acute chest syndrome.

The second publication by Zipursky et al (17) hypothesized that inhalation of 50% oxygen would prevent and reverse erythrocyte sickling. Pain was defined as an acute painful vaso-occlusive crisis. Pain assessment was performed using the McGrath behavioral pain scale with a score of = 6 representing moderate to severe pain. The authors reported a significant reduction in the number of reversible sickled red blood cells in patients who received oxygen. Laboratory evidence of fewer reversible sickled red blood cells did not produce any significant clinical improvements. Patients treated with oxygen therapy had no difference in LOS when compared to room air (6.7 vs 5.4 days, p=NS) or opioid duration (4.7 vs 3.9 days, p=NS).

Transcutaneous electrical nerve stimulation

Many pain management strategies beyond pharmacotherapy exist. Unfortunately, few have been prospectively evaluated in SCD pain. A single study evaluating the use of transcutaneous electrical nerve stimulation (TENS) was identified in the literature search (20). Wang et al (20) hypothesized the use of TENS during an acute SCD-pain episode would produce an improvement in pain scores when compared to a placebo in a double-blind trial. Primary outcomes were pain scores and cumulative opioid use. SCD-pain severity was stratified by the following scale: Grade I or mild pain with pain score 1-4, relief with oral analgesic and no need for hospitalization; Grade II or moderate pain with pain score 5-7, relief with oral analgesic and no need for hospitalization; Grade III or severe pain with pain score 8-10, relief after dose of parenteral opioids, and no need for hospitalization' and Grade

IV or severe pain with pain score 8-10, little or no relief from parenteral opioids and need for hospitalization. Pain was assessed using a 0 to 10 verbal scale. No difference was found in pain scores or amount of adjuvant analgesics required. The authors reported no substantial benefit from the use of TENS at any degree of SCD-pain.

Clinical trials in pain evaluating behavioral interventions

The optimal treatment of pain is multi-modal, combining pharmacotherapy, non-traditional methods, and behavioral interventions. A single trial was identified that prospectively evaluated a pain coping skills intervention in children with SCD (21). In this trial, children were randomized to routine medical care or a coping skills intervention that included deep breathing relaxation, pleasant imagery, and calming self-talk. The primary outcome measures were pain sensitivity, coping strategy use, and clinical measures such as health care utilization and number of school days missed 1-month after intervention. No specific definition of SCD-pain was given. Pain was assessed using a 0-10 numerical scale. The authors reported, based on diary entries, that patients who used their coping strategies on days they experienced pain had fewer health care contacts, less school absences and less disruption of home activities than did those patients not using coping strategies. A major obstacle to widespread use of behavioral interventions is who provides the education about such techniques and how are they reimbursed. Further exploration of non-pharmacologic interventions is important and necessary.

Clinical trials in pain evaluating complimentary alternative medicine

Complimentary alternative medicine, for many patients, is equally important as traditional medicine. A single trial, conducted in Africa, was identified in the review. The authors designed a crossover, double-blind, placebo-controlled, randomized trial to investigate the use of an herbal medication that has been shown to produce anti-sickling effects in vitro called niprisan (22). Treatment with12mg/kg/day of niprisan or equivalent placebo was continued for 6 months and subjects served as their own controls. SCD pain was defined as an acute painful event requiring treatment at a healthcare facility or at home with parenteral opioids, equianalgesic doses of oral opioids, parenteral NSAIDs, or equianalgesic doses of oral NSAIDs. Self-reported pain was not measured. The authors reported that patients taking niprisan experienced less work absence (10.4 vs 19.6 days, $p=0.04$) and fewer days in pain (6.9 vs 22.1, $p<0.001$) than when taking placebo. Adverse events included headache and rash with the niprisan. Rate of hospitalization for pain was low in both groups and the number needed to treat to prevent one hospitalization was 33. However, the number needed to treat to prevent an episode of severe pain was 3. No follow-up trials were identified.

Clinical trials in pain evaluating disease-modifying agents

The primary approach to treating SCD-pain centers on symptomatic therapies rather than the prevention of pain. Medications exist that may alter the natural history of SCD-pain. These medications may decrease the leukocyte count, increase the amount of hemoglobin F or improve or prevent red blood cell dehydration. Trials including children and adolescents with SCD are discussed below; organized by postulated mechanism of action.

Chronic transfusion therapy

Regular blood transfusion therapy with the purpose of keeping the hemoglobin S concentration, commonly less than 30% is used frequently in the treatment of SCD-related morbidities. The benefit of blood transfusion therapy to prevent SCD pain was demonstrated in a secondary analysis for the Stroke Prevention (STOP) trial (18), a trial that successfully established the clinical utility of regular blood transfusion therapy to prevent strokes when a high TCD measurement is detected. The STOP trial was a prospective randomized trial, where one arm received chronic blood transfusion therapy with a goal to keep the hemoglobin S level less than 30% and the second arm was observation (67). A pain episode was defined as pain in the extremities, back, abdomen, chest or head for which no other explanation could be found lasting at least two hours and requiring a medical visit. Self-reported pain was not assessed. No difference in number of pain episodes was found in the intent to treat analysis (16.2 vs 27.1; p=0.13). When patients were analyzed based on actual therapy received, a significant difference was found in frequency of SCD-pain between patients receiving transfusion therapy and standard care (9.7 vs 27.1 events; p = .014). The number needed to treat with chronic transfusion therapy to prevent one episode of pain in the intent to treat analysis was 7. The authors concluded that although chronic transfusion provided a benefit, it was unclear whether the benefits outweighed the significant risks, such as infection, iron overload and allo-immunization, of chronic transfusion therapy. Current clinical practice is varied in the use of chronic blood transfusion to prevent painful episodes. Some sickle cell disease centers will use this strategy after failure to improve with hydroxyurea therapy, while other will not employ such a strategy.

Phlebotomy

A single pilot study was identified evaluating the use of phlebotomy to prevent SCD-pain (19). The authors hypothesized that reduction in hemoglobin would decrease the frequency of hospitalization and performed a prospective, cohort of seven patients. Patients were used as their own historical controls. Primary outcome was number of hospital days. SCD-pain was not formally defined, and pain assessment was not performed. The mean starting hemoglobin was 10.5 gm/dL and was titrated to 8.8-9.2 gm/dl by phlebotomy. The patients were followed for four years after initiation of phlebotomy and the authors report a significant reduction in the number of hospital days (144 to 20, 5, 6 and 1 in the subsequent years). This strategy would only be relevant for patients with elevated steady-state hemoglobin levels, and is not generalizable to most patients with SCD. In addition, lower hematocrit values have been associated with the development of cognitive deficits in children with SCD-Hb SS (68) as well as an increased risk of death, stroke and leg ulcers in the Cooperative Study of Sickle Cell Disease (CSSCD) (69). We can not be sure the benefits of lowering the hemoglobin are better than leaving the patient at the higher hemoglobin and adding hydroxyurea.

Aspirin as an anti-platelet agent

Aspirin may be used as both an analgesic and an anti-platelet agent. Platelet adhesion is thought to play a role in the development of vaso-occlusion in SCD. Two trials were identified that explored the anti-platelet activity of aspirin for the prevention of SCD-pain in children.

The first study was performed in the United States and compared aspirin to a placebo in a double-blind crossover trial (12). Primary outcomes included number of SCD-pain episodes, duration of episode and number of days in pain. SCD-Pain was defined as a VOC and was assessed using a numerical score that included oral versus parenteral analgesics, activity level and number of involved sites. No difference in number of painful episodes (43 vs 49 days, p=NS), duration of painful episode (3.9 vs 3.2 days, p=NS), or total number of days in pain (140 vs 153 days, p=NS) was found between the aspirin and placebo groups. The authors concluded that aspirin did not prevent SCD-pain.

The second study, performed in Brazil, was also a placebo-controlled crossover design and included both children and adults (13). Patients were randomized to receive either 17-45 mg/kg/day of aspirin or a placebo of identical appearing pills. Treatment was continued for 5 months and then each group switched treatment assignments. Patients served as their own controls. SCD-pain was defined as a painful crisis. Pain assessment was not described. No difference in the frequency of SCD-pain was seen between aspirin and placebo treatment periods (40 vs 40 episodes, p=NS). The authors concluded aspirin alone was ineffective in the prevention of SCD-pain.

Hemoglobin F induction

The most well-known inducer of Hemoglobin F production is hydroxyurea. Hydroxyurea has been most extensively studied in adults with SCD-Hb SS. An open-label, single-arm, pilot study was identified assessing the effect of hydroxyurea on pain rate in children and adolescents with SCD (23). Primary outcomes were hemoglobin level, toxicities and frequency of SCD-pain. Patients served as their own controls. SCD-pain was defined as any painful episode involving the extremities, abdomen, back or chest, including ACS that resulted in hospitalization. The authors reported a decrease in mean number of pain episodes, from 2.5 to 0.87 ($p<0.00001$), after starting hydroxyurea therapy. One patient experienced asymptomatic neutropenia; a second, hair loss; a third, excessive nausea, and three patients developed excessively high hemoglobin levels. The number needed to treat with hydroxyurea to prevent one episode of pain was 8. Based on the incidence of neutropenia in this trial, for every 14 patients receiving hydroxyurea, one would develop this potential harm. No other follow-up or long-term studies were located at the time of this review.

Other inhibitors of *in vitro* sickling

Several other medications producing anti-sickling effects in vitro have been described. The review identified five trials assessing the efficacy of four different compounds to prevent pain in children and adolescents with SCD; one study evaluated cromolyn sodium with or without hydroxyurea, one study evaluated piracetam, two studies evaluated poloxamer 188 and one study evaluated pentoxifylline.

Cromolyn sodium

Cromolyn sodium has been hypothesized to have in vitro anti-sickling effects as well as altering neutrophil chemotaxis. A single trial was identified using this modality, a single-blind crossover study of cromolyn sodium with or without hydroxyurea (24). The primary outcome was pain scores and laboratory measurements of sickling. SCD pain was not specifically defined. Pain was assessed using the Wong-Baker FACES scale. The authors reported less in vitro sickling in patients receiving cromolyn sodium and hydroxyurea than cromolyn sodium alone but no difference when compared to patients receiving only hydroxyurea, suggesting any effects were due to hydroxyurea and not cromolyn sodium. Mean number of hospitalizations decreased overall from 3.4 to 2.3 during the study period but no statistical tests were reported and number of hospitalizations was not broken-down by treatment assignment. Pain scores were not different between groups except for patients receiving hydroxyurea plus cromolyn sodium and those receiving cromolyn sodium alone (3.2 vs 5.6; $p = <.05$). The authors concluded patients with mild to moderate SCD should receive cromolyn sodium although pain was not different when compared to placebo and any treatment effect reported was only seen with the addition of hydroxyurea. Evidence of anti-sickling effects on laboratory testing did not correlate with any clinical outcomes.

Piracetam

The next study evaluated the use of piracetam, a dietary supplement, which has been shown to reverse in vitro sickling and decrease endothelial adhesion (25). The authors hypothesized piracetam would be beneficial for children and adolescents with a history of significant SCD-pain and performed a crossover, double-blind, placebo-controlled trial. Primary outcome was difference in monthly pain scores, specific to this study. SCD-pain was defined as a vaso-occlusive crisis in the limbs, vertebral spine, thorax or abdomen, of variable intensity and duration, without other identifiable cause, with or without medical assistance, preferably recognized by patients and relatives as the characteristic pain caused by the disease. Pain was assessed using a visual analog scale (VAS). Monthly pain scores were calculated using pain intensity, duration of pain in days and duration of placebo or piracetam use. The authors found no difference in pain scores between piracetam and placebo (2.1 vs 1.8, $p=0.11$). No further studies of piracetam in SCD were identified.

Poloxamer 188

Two trials of the synthetic compound Poloxamer 188 (PP188) in children and adolescents with SCD-pain were found. PP188 is a non-ionic block copolymer that improves microvascular blood flow by decreasing viscosity and cellular adhesion.

Adams-Graves et al (26) described a phase II, randomized, double-blind, placebo-controlled pilot study evaluating the safety and efficacy of PP188 during an acute SCD-pain episode. Duration of painful episode was the primary efficacy endpoint; analgesic doses, pain intensity and LOS were secondary efficacy endpoints. SCD pain was defined as moderate or severe pain, typical of usual painful event, lasting at least four hours, but not more than 18 hours requiring admission for parenteral analgesics. Pain was assessed with a 5-point 0 to 3 verbal scale. No serious adverse effects were seen; the most common side effect was headache but frequency was not different between groups. Duration of painful episode did not differ between patients receiving PP188 versus placebo (67 vs 80 hrs, $p=0.18$). The authors reported a non-significant decrease in hospital LOS (5 vs 6 days, $p=0.26$); a 3 to 5-fold decrease in median morphine equivalents used (57 vs 159 mg, $p=0.2$); and lower pain intensity scores (0.8 vs 1.4, $p=0.49$) in patients receiving PP188. The authors concluded further trials investigating the efficacy and safety of PP188 were indicated.

In the second publication, also a randomized, double-blind, placebo-controlled trial, the authors hypothesized that PP188 would increase tissue oxygenation, reduce inflammation and pain, and shorten overall length of painful episode in children and adults with SCD-pain (27). The primary outcome was duration of painful episode; secondary outcomes included time to discharge, VAS scores, pain resolution and analgesic consumption. SCD-pain was defined as the sudden onset of acute pain in = 1 sites typical of vaso-occlusive crisis requiring parenteral analgesics. Pain was assessed using a 100-cm visual analog scale (VAS). The authors reported a statistically significant decrease in duration of painful episode in children under 15 years of age receiving PP188 (127 vs 149 hrs, $p<0.01$). Mean morphine equivalents used were not different between groups (0.53 vs 0.72 mg/kg; $p=0.18$). The authors also found no difference in adverse events between groups; no renal complications were noted. The authors concluded that further studies of PP188 were needed especially in children.

Pentoxifylline

A single trial of pentoxifylline in SCD was identified; it was significantly older than the previously discussed trials. Pentoxifylline, commonly used to treat claudication due to peripheral vascular disease, has been shown to improve blood flow and tissue oxygenation. The authors hypothesized the addition of pentoxifylline would improve clinical outcomes in patients with SCD and performed a randomized, double-blind, placebo-controlled trial (28). Treatment duration was six weeks. Primary outcomes included pain intensity, frequency and duration. SCD-pain was divided into three groups: Type A, patients who experience permanent pain in muscles, bones, joints or mixed without fever or other organ involvement; Type B, patients with intermittent pain in muscles, bones, joints or mixed without fever or other organ involvement; and Type C, painful crises in muscles, bones and joints with fever, organ involvement and pronounced hemolysis. Pain intensity was measured using a patient self-report 4-point scale. Patients who received pentoxifylline experienced shorter duration of pain (4.1 vs 8.8 days; $p<0.05$), fewer episodes of pain (57 vs 219; $p<0.05$) and recorded lower pain scores than patients receiving placebo (no statistical tests reported). The author concluded pentoxifylline was a potentially useful medication with minimal adverse effects and warranted further investigation. No other studies have been published in children since this article in 1987.

The assessment of pain in children

Validated, objective measures of pain do not currently exist. As a result, patient self-report has become the best, most reliable measure of pain intensity and pain relief. Pain assessment in children is often more challenging due to developmental variability. Young children do not possess the vocabulary needed to describe pain and also lack the ability to understand abstract concepts required to use numerical or visual pain scales. As a result, the assessment of pain in children requires the use of both observational and behavioral pain scales and self-report pain scales that are properly anchored for the child's developmental stage. In addition, approximately 11% (70) and 20% (71) of the children with sickle cell anemia will have an overt stroke or silent cerebral infarct, respectively. Despite the high prevalence of brain injury among children and adolescents with SCD, pain assessment has never been completed. Thus, traditional assessment of pain may not be applicable to the entire SCD population and will need to be individualized based on pre-established metrics discussed with the parents and the patient as part of the pain action plan.

Behavioral scales

Behavioral and observational scales are important for pre-verbal children, children with alterations in normal developmental and children who are incapacitated such as due to mechanical ventilation. A number of scales were initially developed for post-operative or procedural pain (72). Two scales have been extensively validated and found to have good inter-rater reliability. The Children's Hospital of Eastern Ontario Pain Scale (CHEOPS) has been validated for use in children 4 months to 17 years and has been used in studies of post-operative pain, immunizations, fracture reduction and SCD pain (73). It, however, produces scores that range from 4 to 16, with 4 to 6 indicating no pain. These scores may be difficult to interpret unless the user is highly experienced and are dissonant from the prevailing 5 or 10-point self-report scales. A second scale, the Face, Legs, Arms, Cry, Consolability (FLACC), is an alternative observational scale with equal validity to the CHEOPS, but more easily understood (74). The FLACC scale has been studied in children and adolescents ages 0-18 years and produces scores from 0 to 10 with 0, being no pain and 10, being the most pain. The FLACC has also been shown to have moderate concurrent validity with the FACES pain scale and good concurrent validity with the Visual Analog Scale (VAS). Neither the CHEOPS nor FLACC has been specifically validated for use in children with SCD.

Patient self-report scales

The absence of objective pain measures has increased the importance of self-reported pain. Several different types of self-report scales exist, but the two best suited for the assessment of pain in children are a visual analog scale and a faces-based scale (75). Verbal or verbal numerical pain scales have never been validated for use in children. Visual Analog Scales (VAS) have been extensively investigated and have good validity for children = 8 years (76). Young children tend to choose the extremes of the scales, affecting their interpretation. Although they are quick and easy to use, VAS scales require extensive explanation prior to use in children and adolescents. A wide variety of facial scales have also been developed. The most popular Wong-Baker FACES scale has six faces scoring from 0 to 5, has excellent construct validity, is highly feasible and can be used in children from 3 to 18 years (77).

The FACES scale also requires verbal anchors for the faces; and a smiling, non-neutral "0" face may falsely elevate scores as anxiety associated with medical care or procedures prohibits choosing a smiling face. The FACES scale has become the preferred measure in clinical practice but has lower responsivity to changes in pain which may hamper its use in clinical trials. The Faces pain scale is similar to the Wong-Baker FACES scale except is contains 7 gender-neutral faces scored from 0 to 6 with a non-smiling, neutral "0" face indicating no pain (78). Pain needs to be assessed in two very different ways-in routine clinical care and within clinical trials. The primary goal is often dissimilar in each of these situations. The Faces scale lacks upper-end bias with a neutral face, and is, therefore, better suited for use in clinical trials where the endpoint is generalizing the efficacy of one treatment compared to another to a larger population.

The FACES scale is extremely popularity and one of the most frequently used self-report pain scale in clinical care where the endpoint is response to a patient-specific intervention. Maintaining separate pain scales for use in the clinical care and clinical trial setting may have advantages. The Oucher pain scale combines 6 culturally-sensitive photographic faces with a 100-mm adjacent scale. The Oucher scale has shown good construct and content validity (79). However, the faces are not gender-neutral and their use in young children has not been validated.

The scale is also expensive to reproduce, limiting its use in large-scale clinical and research settings. Given these limitations, this scale is not an appropriate pain scale for young children with sickle cell disease, but would be reasonable for children older than 6 years.

Pain assessment in SCD

Several self-report pain measures have been evaluated for use in children and adolescents with SCD and pain. The Oucher African-American Scale, the Wong-Baker FACES scale and the Visual Analog Scale have been specifically validated in children and adolescents with SCD and pain. In a trial of 100 children ages 3-18 yrs, Luffy et al (80) sought to compare the validity, reliability and preference of these three scales. All three scales proved valid in this patient population. However, the Wong-Baker FACES and Oucher Scales were significantly more reliable than the VAS. Additionally, patients of all ages chose the Wong-Baker FACES scale as their preferred method of pain assessment followed by the Oucher Scale and the VAS.

Pain action plan

The ability to anticipate pre-defined strategies for the treatment of pain is an important component of empowering the patient and the family. Beyer et al (81) performed a qualitative research study to establish the phases or chronology of SCD-pain in children. Eight phases were identified including a prodromal or pre-pain state heralding impending pain (Phase 2); a pain starting point (Phase 3) and a point of pain acceleration (Phase 4) to peak pain (Phase 5). Pain intensity often plateaued at Phase 5 until the point where pain began to decrease (Phase 6) and then steadily declined (Phase 7) until complete resolution (Phase 8) (see figure 2).

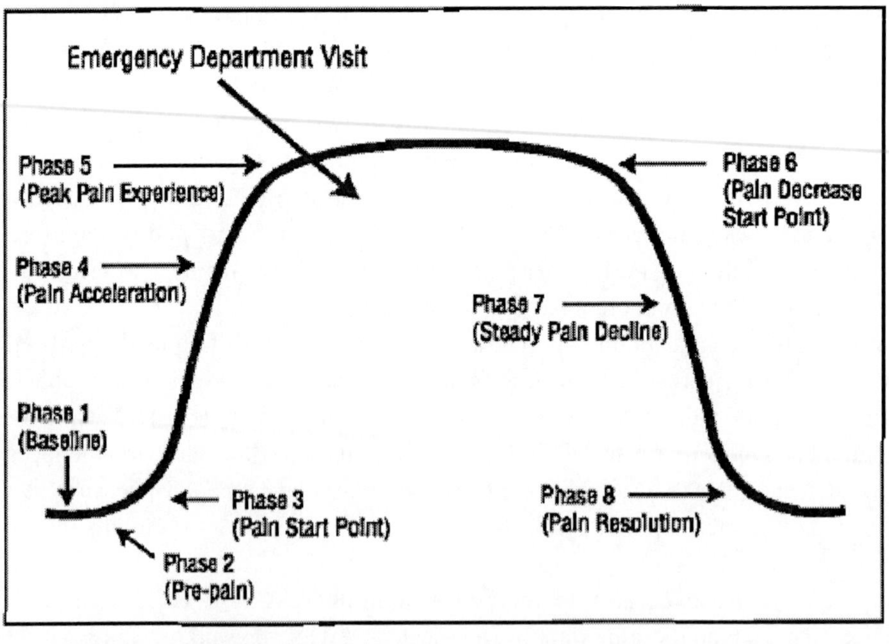

Figure 2 Pain cycle in children with sickle cell disease. From Beyer JE, et al. Arch Pediatr Adolesc Med 1999;153: 913-920 with permission.

Each phase presents a potential target for therapy. Developing an individualized pain action based on these stages of pain can provide the best pain management by combining both pain assessment and flexible treatment depending upon the magnitude of pain. A written pain action plan, given to the patient and caregivers and kept in the medical record, can consistently communicate the next best treatment step based on the level of pain severity for patients, caregivers and healthcare providers.

Study design in pediatric clinical pain trials

The treatment of pain is challenging in all children. Barriers to successful treatment include poorly defined pharmacokinetics of most analgesics in children, practitioner fear of adverse events, and difficulty in assessing responses in pre-verbal children, resulting in the under treatment of pain (82). A need for high-quality clinical trials evaluating the efficacy and safety of analgesics for both children with and without SCD exists. Post-operative pain is the most comprehensively evaluated pain scenario in children. In our literature review, we identified 22 prospective, randomized clinical trials evaluating the use of IV morphine in pediatric post-operative pain to compare primary outcomes, the use of self-report pain assessment (see table 4)(39-60) and study methodology (see table 5) with the SCD pain studies previously discussed.

Table 4. The Use of Validated Self-Report Pain Measures in Pediatric Pain Trials

Method of Pain Measurement	Pediatric Pain Trials (n=22)	SCD Pain Trials (n=27)
VAS	22% (5 [43, 46, 48, 55-56])	37% (10 [6-10, 15, 20-21, 25, 27])
Verbal Numerical Scale	18 % (4 [41, 49, 58, 60])	19% (5 [2, 8, 11, 26, 28])
Wong-Baker FACES Scale or other faces scale	5% (1[45])	11% (3 [3, 7, 24])
Oucher Scale	9% (2 [39, 56])	4% (1 [3])
CHEOPS	18% (4 [39, 49, 52, 56])	4% (1 [3])
Other Behavioral Scales	36% (8 [42, 44-45, 47, 50-51, 53-54])	7% (2 [5, 17])
None used	14% (3 [40, 57, 59])	33% (9 [4, 12-14, 16, 18-19, 22-23])

CHEOPS = Children's Hospital of Eastern Ontario Pain Scale; VAS = Visual Analog Scale.

Methodology

The highest quality of evidence to evaluate the efficacy of pain therapy is a double-blind, placebo-controlled randomized clinical trials. The use of placebo-alone in the treatment of pain in children is unethical. A child experiencing pain must receive an active analgesic and, therefore, most pain clinical trials compare the efficacy between two analgesics or an additional analgesic versus a placebo as adjuvant therapy.

Table 5. Methodologies Used in Post-operative Pediatric Pain Trials Compared to Pediatric SCD Pain Trials

Methodology	Pediatric Pain Trials (n=22)	SCD Pain Trials (n=27)
Self-Report Pain Assessment	45% (10 [39, 41, 43, 46, 48-49, 55-56, 58, 60])	59% (16 [2-3, 6-11, 15, 20-21, 24-28])
Placebo-Controlled	23% (5 [45, 47, 49, 52, 55])	59% (16 [3, 5, 6, 8, 11-15, 20, 22, 24-28])
Double-Blind	77% (17 [39, 44-45, 48-60])	44% (12 [3, 6, 11-12, 14-15, 20, 22, 25-28])
Randomized	100% (22 [39-60])	63% (17 [3, 5, 6, 8-9, 11-15, 17-18, 20-22, 26-28])
Control Group	95% (21 [39-42, 44-45, 46-60])	77% (21 [3, 5, 6, 8-9, 11-18, 20-22, 24-28])
Outcome Measures		
Pain Relief	81% (18 [39, 41, 43-56, 58, 60])	56% (15 [2-4, 7, 9-11, 15, 17, 20, 24-28])
LOS/Duration of Pain	0	44% (12 [4-5, 10, 14-17, 19, 25-28])
Rate of Hospitalization	0	11% (3 [6, 7, 21])
Cumulative Opioid Dose	27% (6 [40, 43, 44-47])	33% (9 [2-3, 5-6, 8, 14-15, 17, 26])
Time to First Analgesia	9% (2 [49, 59])	4% (1 [4])
Clinical Complications	22% (5 [40-41, 45-47])	4% (1 [14])
Physiologic Measure	14% (3 [42-43, 47])	0
Number of Painful Episodes	0	19% (5 [12-13, 18, 22-23])

CHEOPS = Children's Hospital of Eastern Ontario Pain Scale; VAS = Visual Analog Scale; LOS = Length of Stay.

Performing double-blinded randomized trials in acute pain produces other challenges as well. The ability to obtain informed consent or assent during acute pain is difficult, especially if analgesics have already been administered and mental status has been altered. Post-operative pain has the advantage of, in many cases, being predictable and allowing time for consent several days before the operation. Trauma and SCD pain are very unpredictable. Concerns regarding delay of appropriate analgesics while waiting for informed consent, enrollment or randomization assignment are real.

Outcome measures

Given that the etiology and natural history of post-operative pain and SCD pain is quite different, efficacy outcomes commonly used in post-operative pain are not relevant in SCD pain. The most common measures used in SCD pain trials include length of hospital stay (LOS), cumulative opioid dose, and, less frequently, pain relief. The incidence of opioid-induced side effects is also important, but has traditionally been less likely to be noted in the SCD pain trials. Post-operative pain trials in children also include cumulative opioid dose and pain relief. However, rather than focus on LOS, they focus on amount of time between doses or how long to first post-operative analgesia request.

Conclusions

Further investigation of current analgesic regimens employed in SCD-pain in children and adolescents is warranted. Although high quality, double-blind, randomized trials should be a priority, well-designed pharmacokinetic, pharmacodynamic and pharmacogenetics studies are needed. Observational and self-report pain assessment in children and adolescents with SCD-pain are equally important. The more relevant and standardized outcome measures in the assessment of pain for children and adolescents with SCD should be systematically applied to future clinical trials.

References

[1] Smith WR, Penberthy LT, Bovbjerg VE, et al. Daily assessment of pain in adults with sickle cell disease. Ann Intern Med 2008;148(2):94-101.

[2] Christensen ML, Wang WC, Harris S, et al. Transdermal fentanyl administration in children and adolescents with sickle cell pain crisis. J Pediatr Hematol Oncol 1996;18(4):372-6.

[3] Jacobson SJ, Kopecky EA, Joshi P, et al. Randomised trial of oral morphine for painful episodes of sickle-cell disease in children. Lancet 1997;350(9088):1358-61.

[4] Melzer-Lange MD, Walsh-Kelly CM, Lea G, et al. Patient-controlled analgesia for sickle cell pain crisis in a pediatric emergency department. Pediatr Emerg Care 2004;20(1):2-4.

[5] Robieux IC, Kellner JD, Coppes MJ, et al. Analgesia in children with sickle cell crisis: comparison of intermittent opioids vs. continuous intravenous infusion of morphine and placebo-controlled study of oxygen inhalation. Pediatr Hematol Oncol 1992;9(4):317-26.

[6] Hardwick WE, Jr., Givens TG, Monroe KW, et al. Effect of ketorolac in pediatric sickle cell vaso-occlusive pain crisis. Pediatr Emerg Care 1999;15(3):179-82.
[7] Beiter JL, Jr., Simon HK, Chambliss CR, et al. Intravenous ketorolac in the emergency department management of sickle cell pain and predictors of its effectiveness. Arch Pediatr Adolesc Med 2001;155(4):496-500.
[8] Perlin E, Finke H, Castro O, et al. Enhancement of pain control with ketorolac tromethamine in patients with sickle cell vaso-occlusive crisis. Am J Hematol 1994;46(1):43-7.
[9] Grisham JE VE. Ketorolac versus meperidine in vaso-occlusive crisis: a study of safety and efficacy. Int J Pediatr Hematol Oncol 1996;3:239-47.
[10] de Franceschi L, Finco G, Vassanelli A, et al. A pilot study on the efficacy of ketorolac plus tramadol infusion combined with erythrocytapheresis in the management of acute severe vaso-occlusive crises and sickle cell pain. Haematologica 2004;89(11):1389-91.
[11] Eke FU, Obamyonyi A, Eke NN, et al. An open comparative study of dispersible piroxicam versus soluble acetylsalicylic acid for the treatment of osteoarticular painful attack during sickle cell crisis. Trop Med Int Health 2000;5(2):81-4.
[12] Greenberg J, Ohene-Frempong K, Halus J, et al. Trial of low doses of aspirin as prophylaxis in sickle cell disease. J Pediatr 1983;102(5):781-4.
[13] Zago MA, Costa FF, Ismael SJ, et al. Treatment of sickle cell diseases with aspirin. Acta Haematol 1984;72(1):61-4.
[14] Griffin TC, McIntire D, Buchanan GR. High-dose intravenous methylprednisolone therapy for pain in children and adolescents with sickle cell disease. N Engl J Med 1994;330(11):733-7.
[15] Weiner DL, Hibberd PL, Betit P, et al. Preliminary assessment of inhaled nitric oxide for acute vaso-occlusive crisis in pediatric patients with sickle cell disease. JAMA 2003;289(9):1136-42.
[16] Brousseau DC, Scott JP, Hillery CA, et al. The effect of magnesium on length of stay for pediatric sickle cell pain crisis. Acad Emerg Med 2004;11(9):968-72.
[17] Zipursky A, Robieux IC, Brown EJ, et al. Oxygen therapy in sickle cell disease. Am J Pediatr Hematol Oncol 1992;14(3):222-8.
[18] Miller ST, Wright E, Abboud M, et al. Impact of chronic transfusion on incidence of pain and acute chest syndrome during the Stroke Prevention Trial (STOP) in sickle-cell anemia. J Pediatr 2001;139(6):785-9.
[19] Bouchair N, Manigne P, Kanfer A, et al. [Prevention of sickle cell crises with multiple phlebotomies]. Arch Pediatr 2000;7(3):249-55.
[20] Wang WC, George SL, Wilimas JA. Transcutaneous electrical nerve stimulation treatment of sickle cell pain crises. Acta Haematol 1988;80(2):99-102.
[21] Gil KM, Anthony KK, Carson JW, et al. Daily coping practice predicts treatment effects in children with sickle cell disease. J Pediatr Psychol 2001;26(3):163-73.
[22] Wambebe COBE, Badru BO, Khamofu H, Momoh JA, Ekpeyong E, et al. Efficacy of niprisan in the prophylactic management of patients with sickle cell disease. Curr Ther Res Clin Exp 2000:62(1):26-34.
[23] Jayabose S, Tugal O, Sandoval C, et al. Clinical and hematologic effects of hydroxyurea in children with sickle cell anemia. J Pediatr 1996;129(4):559-65.
[24] Karimi M, Zekavat OR, Sharifzadeh S, et al. Clinical response of patients with sickle cell anemia to cromolyn sodium nasal spray. Am J Hematol 2006;81(11):809-16.
[25] Alvim RC, Viana MB, Pires MA, et al. Inefficacy of piracetam in the prevention of painful crises in children and adolescents with sickle cell disease. Acta Haematol 2005;113(4):228-33.
[26] Adams-Graves P, Kedar A, Koshy M, et al. RheothRx (poloxamer 188) injection for the acute painful episode of sickle cell disease: a pilot study. Blood 1997;90(5):2041-6.
[27] Orringer EP, Casella JF, Ataga KI, et al. Purified poloxamer 188 for treatment of acute vaso-occlusive crisis of sickle cell disease: A randomized controlled trial. JAMA 2001;286(17):2099-2106.

[28] Manrique RV. Placebo controlled double-blind study of pentoxifylline in sickle cell disease patients. J Med 1987;18(5-6):277-91.

[29] Buchanan ID, Woodward M, Reed GW. Opioid selection during sickle cell pain crisis and its impact on the development of acute chest syndrome. Pediatr Blood Cancer 2005;45(5):716-24.

[30] Carbajal R, Hubert P, Treluyer JM, et al. Nitrous oxide and morphine in children with sickle cell crisis. Lancet 1996;347(9015):1621.

[31] Holbrook CT. Patient-controlled analgesia pain management for children with sickle cell disease. J Assoc Acad Minor Phys 1990;1(3):93-6.

[32] Huehns ER, Davies SC, Brozovic M. Fresh frozen plasma for vaso-occlusive crises in sickle cell disease. Lancet 1981;1(8233):1310-1.

[33] Kopecky EA, Jacobson S, Joshi P, et al. Systemic exposure to morphine and the risk of acute chest syndrome in sickle cell disease. Clin Pharmacol Ther 2004;75(3):140-6.

[34] Schechter NL, Berrien FB, Katz SM. The use of patient-controlled analgesia in adolescents with sickle cell pain crisis: a preliminary report. J Pain Symptom Manage 1988;3(2):109-13.

[35] Styles LA, Vichinsky E. Effects of a long-term transfusion regimen on sickle cell-related illnesses. J Pediatr 1994;125(6 Pt 1):909-11.

[36] Trentadue NO, Kachoyeanos MK, Lea G. A comparison of two regimens of patient-controlled analgesia for children with sickle cell disease. J Pediatr Nurs 1998;13(1):15-9.

[37] Woods GM, Parson PM, Strickland DK. Efficacy of nalbuphine as a parenteral analgesic for the treatment of painful episodes in children with sickle cell disease. J Assoc Acad Minor Phys 1990;1(3):90-2.

[38] Yaster M, Tobin JR, Billett C, et al. Epidural analgesia in the management of severe vaso-occlusive sickle cell crisis. Pediatrics 1994;93(2):310-5.

[39] Lieh-Lai MW, Kauffman RE, Uy HG, et al. A randomized comparison of ketorolac tromethamine and morphine for postoperative analgesia in critically ill children. Crit Care Med 1999;27(12):2786-91.

[40] Mather SJ, Peutrell JM. Postoperative morphine requirements, nausea and vomiting following anaesthesia for tonsillectomy. Comparison of intravenous morphine and non-opioid analgesic techniques. Paediatr Anaesth 1995;:5(3):185-8.

[41] Vetter TR. Pediatric patient-controlled analgesia with morphine versus meperidine. J Pain Symptom Manage 1992;7(4):204-8.

[42] Semsroth M, Hiesmayr M. [Continuous application of morphine is more effective than a bolus administration in the postoperative analgesia and sedation of children]. Anaesthesist 1990;39(10):552-6.

[43] McNeely JK, Trentadue NC. Comparison of patient-controlled analgesia with and without nighttime morphine infusion following lower extremity surgery in children. J Pain Symptom Manage 1997;13(5):268-73.

[44] Maunuksela EL, Kokki H, Bullingham RE. Comparison of intravenous ketorolac with morphine for postoperative pain in children. Clin Pharmacol Ther 1992;52(4):436-43.

[45] Sutters KA, Shaw BA, Gerardi JA, et al. Comparison of morphine patient-controlled analgesia with and without ketorolac for postoperative analgesia in pediatric orthopedic surgery. Am J Orthop 1999;28(6):351-8.

[46] Vetter TR, Heiner EJ. Intravenous ketorolac as an adjuvant to pediatric patient-controlled analgesia with morphine. J Clin Anesth 1994;6(2):110-3.

[47] van den Berg AA, Honjol NM, Prabhu NV, et al. Analgesics and ENT surgery. A clinical comparison of the intraoperative, recovery and postoperative effects of buprenorphine, diclofenac, fentanyl, morphine, nalbuphine, pethidine and placebo given intravenously with induction of anaesthesia. Br J Clin Pharmacol 1994;38(6):533-43.

[48] Jylli L, Lundeberg S, Langius-Eklof A, et al. Comparison of the analgesic efficacy of ketobemidone and morphine for management of postoperative pain in children: a randomized, controlled study. Acta Anaesthesiol Scand 2004;48(10):1256-9.

[49] Umuroglu T, Eti Z, Ciftci H, et al. Analgesia for adenotonsillectomy in children: a comparison of morphine, ketamine and tramadol. Paediatr Anaesth 2004;14(7):568-73.

[50] Suresh S, Barcelona SL, Young NM, et al. Postoperative pain relief in children undergoing tympanomastoid surgery: is a regional block better than opioids? Anesth Analg 2002;94(4):859-62.

[51] Purday JP, Reichert CC, Merrick PM. Comparative effects of three doses of intravenous ketorolac or morphine on emesis and analgesia for restorative dental surgery in children. Can J Anaesth 1996;43(3):221-5.

[52] Weinstein MS, Nicolson SC, Schreiner MS. A single dose of morphine sulfate increases the incidence of vomiting after outpatient inguinal surgery in children. Anesthesiology 1994;81(3):572-7.

[53] Munro HM, Riegger LQ, Reynolds PI, et al. Comparison of the analgesic and emetic properties of ketorolac and morphine for paediatric outpatient strabismus surgery. Br J Anaesth 1994;72(6):624-8.

[54] Wolf AR, Hughes D. Pain relief for infants undergoing abdominal surgery: comparison of infusions of i.v. morphine and extradural bupivacaine. Br J Anaesth 1993;70(1):10-6.

[55] Watcha MF, Jones MB, Lagueruela RG, et al. Comparison of ketorolac and morphine as adjuvants during pediatric surgery. Anesthesiology 1992;76(3):368-72.

[56] Berde CB, Beyer JE, Bournaki MC, et al. Comparison of morphine and methadone for prevention of postoperative pain in 3- to 7-year-old children. J Pediatr 1991;119(1 (Pt 1)):136-41.

[57] Maunuksela EL, Korpela R, Olkkola KT. Comparison of buprenorphine with morphine in the treatment of postoperative pain in children. Anesth Analg 1988:67(3):233-9.

[58] Maunuksela EL, Korpela R, Olkkola KT. Double-blind, multiple-dose comparison of buprenorphine and morphine in postoperative pain of children. Br J Anaesth 1988;60(1):48-55.

[59] Krane EJ, Jacobson LE, Lynn AM, et al. Caudal morphine for postoperative analgesia in children: a comparison with caudal bupivacaine and intravenous morphine. Anesth Analg 1987;66(7):647-53.

[60] Engelhardt T, Steel E, Johnston G, et al. Tramadol for pain relief in children undergoing tonsillectomy: a comparison with morphine. Paediatr Anaesth 2003;13(3):249-52.

[61] Dampier C, Ely E, Brodecki D, et al. Home management of pain in sickle cell disease: a daily diary study in children and adolescents. J Pediatr Hematol Oncol 2002;24(8):643-7.

[62] Prescilla RP, Frattarelli DA, Haritos D, et al. Pharmacokinetics of rofecoxib in children with sickle cell hemoglobinopathy. J Pediatr Hematol Oncol 2004;26(10):661-4.

[63] Frei-Jones MJ, Baxter AL, Rogers ZR, et al. Vaso-occlusive episodes in older children with sickle cell disease: emergency department management and pain assessment. J Pediatr 2008;152(2):281-5.

[64] Simckes AM, Chen SS, Osorio AV, et al. Ketorolac-induced irreversible renal failure in sickle cell disease: a case report. Pediatr Nephrol 1999;13(1):63-7.

[65] DeBaun M. Fatal gastric hemorrhage in an adolescent patient with sickle cell anemia treated with ketorolac and ibuprofen. Unpublished data.

[66] Bernini JC, Rogers ZR, Sandler ES, et al. Beneficial effect of intravenous dexamethasone in children with mild to moderately severe acute chest syndrome complicating sickle cell disease. Blood 1998:92(9);3082-9.

[67] Adams RJ, McKie VC, Hsu L, et al. Prevention of a first stroke by transfusions in children with sickle cell anemia and abnormal results on transcranial Doppler ultrasonography. N Engl J Med 1998;339(1):5-11.

[68] Steen RG, Miles MA, Helton KJ, et al. Cognitive impairment in children with hemoglobin SS sickle cell disease: relationship to MR imaging findings and hematocrit. AJNR Am J Neuroradiol 2003;24(3):382-9.

[69] Quinn CT, Miller ST. Risk factors and prediction of outcomes in children and adolescents who have sickle cell anemia. Hematol Oncol Clin North Am 2004;18(6):1339-54.

[70] Ohene-Frempong K, Weiner SJ, Sleeper LA, et al. Cerebrovascular accidents in sickle cell disease: rates and risk factors. Blood 1998;91(1):288-94.

[71] Armstrong FD, Thompson RJ, Jr., Wang W, et al. Cognitive functioning and brain magnetic resonance imaging in children with sickle Cell disease. Neuropsychology Committee of the Cooperative Study of Sickle Cell Disease. Pediatrics 1996;97(6 Pt 1):864-70.

[72] von Baeyer CL, Spagrud LJ. Systematic review of observational (behavioral) measures of pain for children and adolescents aged 3 to 18 years. Pain 2007;127(1-2):140-50.

[73] McGrath P, Johnson G, Goodman J, et al. CHEOPS: a behavioral scale for rating post-operative pain in children. Adv Pain Research Therapy 1985;9:395-402.

[74] Merkel SI, Voepel-Lewis T, Shayevitz JR, et al. The FLACC: a behavioral scale for scoring postoperative pain in young children. Pediatr Nurs 1997;23(3):293-7.

[75] Stinson JN, Kavanagh T, Yamada J, et al. Systematic review of the psychometric properties, interpretability and feasibility of self-report pain intensity measures for use in clinical trials in children and adolescents. Pain 2006;125(1-2):143-57.

[76] Champion G, Goodenough B, von Baeyer C, et al. Measurement of Pain in Infants and Children. Seattle: IASP Press, 1998.

[77] Wong DL, Baker CM. Pain in children: comparison of assessment scales. Pediatr Nurs 1988;14(1):9-17.

[78] Bieri D, Reeve RA, Champion GD, et al. The Faces Pain Scale for the self-assessment of the severity of pain experienced by children: development, initial validation, and preliminary investigation for ratio scale properties. Pain 1990;41(2):139-150.

[79] Beyer JE, Aradine CR. Content validity of an instrument to measure young children's perceptions of the intensity of their pain. J Pediatr Nurs 1986;1(6):386-95.

[80] Luffy R, Grove SK. Examining the validity, reliability, and preference of three pediatric pain measurement tools in African-American children. Pediatr Nurs 2003;29(1):54-9.

[81] Beyer JE, Simmons LE, Woods GM, et al. A chronology of pain and comfort in children with sickle cell disease. Arch Pediatr Adolesc Med 1999;153(9):913-20.

[82] Walco GA, Cassidy RC, Schechter NL. Pain, hurt, and harm. The ethics of pain control in infants and children. N Engl J Med 1994;331(8):541-4.

In: Children and Pain
Editors: P. Schofield and J. Merrick
ISBN 978-1-60876-020-6

Chapter 10

Sickle cell disease: Guidelines for treatment of pain in hospitalized children

***Melissa J Frei-Jones, MD*[*1,2] and Michael R DeBaun, MD MPH*[2,3]**
[1]Department of Pediatrics, Washington University School of Medicine, St Louis, Missouri
[2]Hematology-Oncology, Department of Pediatrics, University of Texas Health Science Center, San Antonio, Texas
[3]Department of Genetics, Washington University School of Medicine, St Louis, Missouri, United States of America

Abstract

Pain is the most common morbidity experienced by children with sickle cell disease (SCD). When outpatient pain management strategies fail, two-thirds of patients seen in the emergency department (ED) will ultimately require inpatient admission. Many of the common strategies used to treat hospitalized children with vaso-occlusive pain episodes are based on available clinical evidence and experience; limited practical guidelines exist for the inpatient management of pain in SCD. We identified supporting evidence for the use of selected opioid analgesics, scheduled intravenous (IV) pain medications, patient controlled analgesia (PCA), weaning from maximum dose with conversion to equianalgesic oral pain medications, and use of incentive spirometry during inpatient management of acute painful episodes. Despite the perception of the benefit, no evidence could be identified and limited to no expert opinion supported the use of rapid infusion of intravenous (IV) fluids (boluses), blood transfusions, prophylactic oxygen, antihistamine therapy, and ketorolac or methadone administration for the management of acute SCD pain. In several instances, significant toxicities have been identified with these therapies that have marginal to no proven benefit for the treatment of inpatient

[*] Correspondence: Assistant Professor Melissa Frei-Jones, MD, Msci, Hematology-Oncology, Department of Pediatrics, University of Texas Health Science Center, 333 N. Santa Rosa, RM B8208, San Antonio, TX 78207 United States. E-mail: FreiJones@uthscsa.edu

painful episodes in children with SCD. Establishing a standard pain management strategy that is consistent, transparent and easy to follow is an important for optimal inpatient management of pain among children with SCD. Clinical strategies that accentuate treatment with a firm pharmacological basis and eliminating therapy that has no proven efficacy will ultimately improve the quality of care for this vulnerable patient population.

Introduction

Pain is the most frequent disease-related complication requiring hospital admission for children with sickle cell disease (SCD). As many as two-thirds of children with SCD who seek emergency department (ED) care for pain will need inpatient treatment leading to over 20,000 discharges annually (1,2). Despite the high prevalence, few evidence-based guidelines or consensus statements exist regarding the inpatient management of painful episodes among children with SCD.

Effective pain management education is inadequate in many medical schools (3) and lack of education produces inadequate pain treatment (4). Practitioners may have preconceived beliefs regarding SCD pain and opioid-seeking behavior. Although the actual rate of true addiction to opioids among children with SCD is less than 1%(5), the prevalence is reported to be much higher by resident physicians and nurses, 17% and 13% respectively (6). The difference in perception and reality in the prevalence of addiction may influence the management of children hospitalized for pain.

Guidelines or clinical pathways have been created in an effort to improve the care of children with SCD. However, the implementation and dissemination of evidence-based guidelines is not straightforward. Barriers exist to changing clinical practice such as failure to provide clear and practical information, personal beliefs and reliance on experience over evidence (7). In addition, research is lacking in the science of implementation and behavioral change. Studies evaluating single interventions or education-only interventions failed to produce improved patient care or adherence to evidence-based guidelines. Multi-interventional studies were more successful but required educational materials, reminders, patient-focused interventions and feedback or audits (8).

In this review, we describe a practical and when available evidence-based pain management strategy for children with SCD and pain requiring hospital treatment.

Sickle cell disease

Accurate communication between house staff, nurses and attending or consulting physicians is important in the care of children with SCD. SCD encompasses multiple inherited disorders of hemoglobin (Hb) synthesis. Clinical classification of these disorders is based on the underlying mutation in the beta (ß) or alpha (α) globin gene. The sickle cell mutation derives from a single base-pair change at the sixth codon of the ß-globin gene cluster on chromosome 11 producing an abnormal protein. Sickle cell anemia (SCA) or homozygous SS (SCD-HbSS) disease results from the presence of the sickle cell mutation in both copies of the ß-globin genes. Compound heterozygotes carry the sickle cell mutation on one ß-globin gene and a second distinct mutation on the other ß-globin gene such as Hb C, Hb ß thalassemia or other rarer variants. The most frequent compound heterozygotes are heterozygous Hb SC (SCD-Hb SC), Hb Sß-thalassemia plus (SCD-Sß+) or Sß-thalassemia null (SCD-Sß°). The specific type of SCD predicts phenotype, baseline laboratory tests, as well as the frequency of SCD-related morbidities such as stroke, acute chest syndrome and pain episodes (9).

SCD affects 72,000 Americans with one in four African-Americans being a carrier of sickle cell trait (SCT). All fifty states participate in newborn screening, begun in 1987 by the National Institutes of Health (NIH), which identifies 2,000 infants annually (10). Clinical research efforts have dramatically improved care through the use of penicillin prophylaxis, hydroxyurea and chronic transfusion therapy (9). Life expectancy for children with SCD-Hb SS has doubled since passage of the National Sickle Cell Anemia Control Act in 1972(11). A 2004 analysis of a newborn SCD cohort found 85% of children survived to 18 years (12).

Acute pain in SCD

A painful episode due to SCD, also termed a vaso-occlusive episode (VOE), is the most common morbidity faced by children and adults with SCD (13). In 1991, the Cooperative Study of Sickle Cell Disease (CSSCD) published the results of a longitudinal study of children and adults with SCD. On average patients with SCD-Hb SS experienced one pain episode per year requiring hospital-based care with 39% having no pain episodes. Additionally, 5% of patients had multiple visits (3-10/year) and comprised 33% of painful episodes. These results illustrate the heterogeneity in the painful episode rate within individual patients (14).

The incidence of painful episodes in SCD is primarily age dependent (14). Classically, the first painful condition seen in infants and young children with SCD is dactylitis or the Hand-Foot Syndrome which is the unilateral, acute painful swelling of the dorsal hands and feet (15). As children become older, the frequency of pain due to vaso-occlusion increases (see figure 1). In the CSSCD, the pain rate for children ages 15-19 years was the same as young adults aged 20-24 and twice the rate seen in children aged 5-9 years (14).

A common pain episode in children with SCD can be defined as the abrupt, episodic onset of pain with no other identifiable cause. In their own words, patients with SCD describe the pain as “knives in my chest” or “like I’m drowning in pain” (16,17). The pain may be localized to the extremities, involve the whole body or visceral organs such as spleen or liver. Pain may be accompanied by localized swelling, decreased mobility, warmth and low-grade fever. Patients may also experience increased hemolysis reflected in scleral icterus and falling hemoglobin levels (15). Jacobs et al (18) further characterized pain episodes in hospitalized children. On average, patients began having pain 4.5 days prior to presentation and two-thirds described the pain as continuous (18). The average length of stay (LOS) for children hospitalized for pain is 4.4 days (19). Some children report no change in pain intensity during hospitalization, but rather a progressive decrease in the surface area of pain (18). Children in pain experienced significant disruptions in sleep patterns and were more likely to miss school while they were having pain(20). In summary, pain is a major complication for children with

SCD-Hb SS that impairs not only their daily activities, but may also account for a high school absence rate (21).

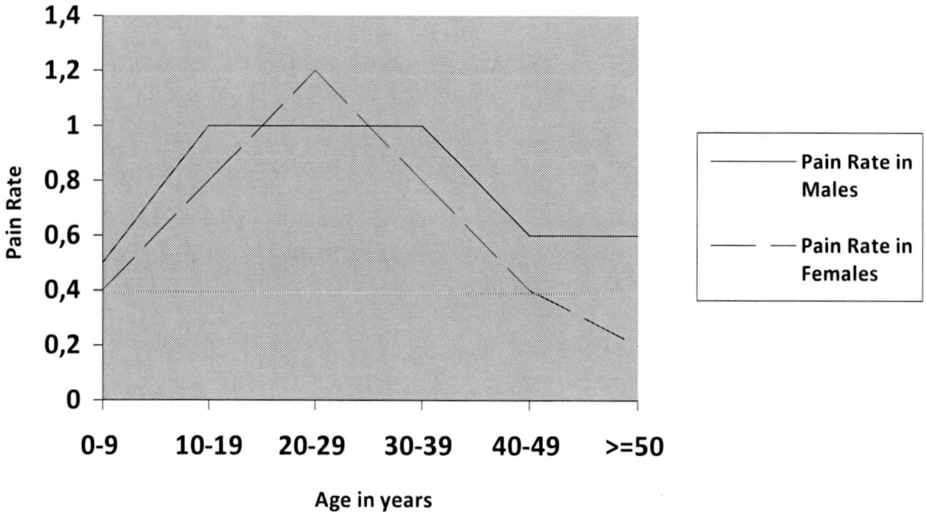

Figure 1. Age-specific pain rates (adapted from N Engl J Med 1991; 325:11-6 with permission).

Risk factors for pain

The pathophysiology of vaso-occlusive pain has not yet been thoroughly described, however it is believed in part to be an inflammatory process (15). The ß-globin gene containing the sickle mutation produces an unstable hemoglobin that has a tendency to polymerize in its deoxygenated state, such as occurs in the tissues where oxygen extraction is more robust. The deoxygenated, polymerized hemoglobin causes red blood cells to change conformation from a flexible bi-concave disc to a sickle-shaped cell. Red blood cells that are sickled in shape cannot move normally through the circulation and result in microvascular occlusion. This vaso-occlusion produces local tissue hypoxia producing tissue damage and inflammation leading to pain.

Pain episodes may occur in isolation or in association with other conditions. They may be precipitated by prolonged swimming, emotional stress, physical exertion, or infection (22-25). Clinical experiments of hand immersion in cool water (16°C) found adults with SCD-Hb SS experienced increasing vasoconstriction and pain with each successive immersion when compared to patients without SCD (26). Temporally, pain often begins or worsens in the late afternoon and evening (24), and frequency of ED visits increases as ambient temperatures fall below 32°C (27). Patients with SCD-Hb SS and co-morbid asthma have a higher rate of pain episodes and acute chest syndrome events than patients without asthma (addboyd, macklin paper) (28,29) (see table 1).

Table 1. Factors associated with the onset of pain in sickle cell disease-Hb SS

1. Swimming in cold water
2. Exercise or physical exertion
3. Infection
4. Change in the ambient temperature below 32°C
5. Emotional stress
6. Menstruation
7. Pregnancy

Phases of pain

Clear understanding of the progression from earliest symptoms to pain resolution is important in successful treatment design. No distinct physiological or biochemical marker for the basis of pain exists. However, a qualitative research study established eight phases of a pain in children (see table 2).

Table 2. Summary of the chronology of pain in children with sickle cell disease. Adapted from Arch Pediatr Adolesc Med 1999;153:913-920

Phase	Pain Characteristics	Suggested Comfort Measures Used
1 (Baseline)	No vaso-occlusive pain; pain of complications may be present, such as that connected with avascular necrosis of the hip.	No measures needed.
2 (Pre-pain)	No vaso-occlusive pain; pain of complications may be present; prodromal signs of impending vaso-occlusive episode may appear, eg. "yellow eyes" and/or fatigue.	No measures used; caregivers may encourage child to increase fluids to prevent pain event from occurring.
3 (Pain start point)	First signs of vaso-occlusive pain appear, usually in mild form.	Mild oral analgesics often given; fluids increased; child usually maintains normal activities.
4 (Pain acceleration)	Intensity of pain increases from mild to moderate. Some children may skip this level or move quickly from phase 3 to phase 5.	Stronger oral analgesics are given; rubbing, heat, or other activities are often used; child usually stays in school until pain becomes more severe, then stays home and limits activities; is usually in bed; family searches for ways to control pain.
5 (Peak pain experience)	Pain accelerates to high moderate or severe levels and plateaus; pain may remain elevated for extended period of time. Child's appearance, behavior, mood are significantly different from normal.	Oral analgesics are given around the clock at home; combinations of comfort measures are used; family may avoid going to the hospital; if pain is so distressing to the child, parent will take the child to the emergency department.

Table 2. (Continued)

Phase	Pain Characteristics	Suggested Comfort Measures Used
		After child enters hospital, families often turn over comforting activities to health care providers and wait to see if the analgesics work. Family caregivers are often tired from exhaustion of caring for the child for several days with little or no rest.
6 (Pain decrease start point)	Pain finally begins to decrease in intensity from the peak pain level.	Family caregivers again become active in comforting the child but not as intensely as during phases 4 and 5.
7 (Steady pain decline)	Pain decreases more rapidly, becoming more tolerable for child. Child and family are more relaxed.	Health care providers begin to wean the child from the intravenous analgesic; oral opioids given; discharge planning is started. Children may be discharged before they are pain free.
8 (Pain resolution)	Pain intensity is at a tolerable level, and discharge is imminent. Child looks and acts like "normal" self. Mood improves.	May receive oral analgesics.

Each of these phases are potential areas for intervention during an episode. Beyer et al (30) identified a prodromal or pre-pain state heralding impending pain (Phase 2). Once pain started, the amount of time to reach peak pain was different for each child. After peaking, pain remained steady before beginning to decrease. The duration and timing of each phase differs between individual patients and between episodes for the same patient challenging the notion of a "typical" pain episode (30). Patients and caregivers can be taught to use the phases as a cue to initiate a pain action plan and escalate care following the plan.

Treatment of acute sickle cell pain

Pain action plan

The most appropriate pain management combines both the accurate assessment of pain with a flexible treatment strategy based on the magnitude of pain. An individualized pain action plan can provide clear communication of the next appropriate treatment step based on the level of pain severity for patients, caregivers and healthcare providers. Such models have been created for the treatment asthma and are useful in improving care (31). For each phase of pain, a treatment strategy should be implemented (see table 1 and appendix 3).

Following a pain action plan requires the regular assessment of pain before and after intervention. Several pain assessment tools have been validated for use in children with SCD and pain. The Wong-Baker FACES Scale, the Oucher African-American Scale and the visual analog scale (VAS) are among the scales most commonly used. When children with SCD were asked which pain scale they preferred, the majority chose the Wong-Baker FACES Scale (32) (see figure 2). A verbal analog scale has not been validated in children with SCD.

0
NO HURT
1
HURTS
LITTLE BIT
2
HURTS
LITTLE MORE
3
HURTS
EVEN MORE
4
HURTS
WHOLE LOT
5
HURTS
WORST

Figure 2. Wong-Baker FACES Pain Rating Scale. From Hockenberry MJ, Wilson D, Winkelstein ML. Wong's essentials of pediatric nursing, 7th ed. St. Louis, MO: Mosby, 2005:1259. Used with permission.

Treating pain at home

The primary basis for pain treatment at home requires an understanding of the pain phases with pre-planned treatment strategies for each stage of pain. For phase 1, no treatment is required as the child is not experiencing acute pain. For phase 2, the prodromal phase where warning signs of impending pain begin to appear, comfort measures should be used such as listening to music, meditation or other non-medicinal strategies. Phase 3 heralds the onset of pain where patients and caregivers should initiate scheduled oral analgesics specific to the child's age and past history of pain. In general, infants and younger children can often be treated with ibuprofen and acetaminophen-codeine combinations for mild to moderate pain. Stronger opioids such as oxycodone and morphine-immediate release (MSIR) are usually reserved for older children, usually greater than five-years of age. Although oxycodone is available in oral preparation, long-acting opioids can only be given as pills and are, therefore, not helpful in younger children. Pharmacokinetics of oxycodone have been described in children but not patients with SCD (33). Oxycontin, the extended release form of oxycodone, may be especially useful due to its favorable pharmacokinetic profile, namely rapid onset. Onset of analgesia for oxycontin occurs within 30-minutes similar to oxycodone. Unlike oxycodone, oxycontin will maintain serum levels for up to 12 hours, providing improved relief and should be given first with the onset of a pain episode in older children. Oxycodone may be given intermittently for periods of sudden increased pain also called breakthrough pain. Older patients and families should try scheduled long-acting analgesics with the use of short-acting analgesics for breakthrough pain and non-medicinal strategies to relieve pain.

Emergency department management

During phase 3 or 4, as pain progresses, patients and their caregivers may present to the outpatient clinic or ED for further pain management. In the ED, the general approach to SCD pain involves excluding non-sickle cell causes of pain, the placement of an intravenous line (IV), laboratory tests such as complete blood count and reticulocyte count, and the administration of IV opioids. The American Pain Society has published algorithms for IV opioid titration (34). Although practices vary between institutions, patients who require two or more doses of IV opioids are usually admitted for further pain management (35). In situations where the patient has not taken any oral opioids prior to ED presentation, the ED staff may initiate oxycontin first because of its rapid onset of analgesia and its sustained effects.

Inpatient pain management

Most patients who present to the ED with severe SCD-related pain will require hospital admission, and admission to the hospital is an indication for scheduled opioids. Thus, there is little advantage in keeping a child in the ED for prolonged periods of time using intermittent IV opioid therapy with the belief that we will decrease the painful episode sufficiently to allow for discharge home.

Opioid type, dose and administration form will vary based on the individual patient, but should be consistent for each patient. Once admitted, children should receive scheduled analgesics for the duration of their pain episode. Young children are frequently treated with intermittent, scheduled IV morphine sulfate. For older children, the use of patient-controlled analgesia (PCA) has become standard care (36-38). Previous research has established that cognitively normal children as young as five years can be taught how to use a PCA (39). Such limits have not been evaluated in children with SCD where 30% of patients will have had a silent or overt cerebral vascular event by their 18th birthday, affecting learning and cognition (40). The ability to successfully use a PCA will vary and necessitates that patients be instructed to identify cues for escalating pain, understand when to self-administer PCA doses and have a proper expectation for time to relief. Patients should also receive adjuvant therapy such as ibuprofen or acetaminophen as recommended by the World Health Organization Pain Ladder if not contraindicated (41) (see appendix 1, 4 and 5).

Choice of analgesic

Morphine sulfate is the most common opioid used in the treatment of SCD painful episodes. Morphine is the only opioid with pharmacokinetics described specifically in children with SCD-Hb SS and these studies demonstrated a significantly higher plasma clearance rate for morphine (42). For treatment purposes, the results in general indicate the same dose of morphine will result in lower plasma levels in a patient with SCD-HbSS compared to a patient without SCD. Additionally, interval increases in dose will not achieve the same rise in serum levels and therefore produces smaller incremental increases in pain relief.

Fentanyl and Hydromorphone are used less frequently. The pharmacokinetics in patients with SCD-Hb SS have not been described for either fentanyl or hydromorphone. A study investigating the use of a fentanyl patch for acute pain found no decrease in supplemental morphine use by PCA or lower pain scores (43). No specific studies of hydromorphone in children have been published. In adults, the use of hydromorphone instead of meperidine in the ED resulted in fewer ED returns and increased utilization of outpatient programs (44). Most often, an alternative opioid is chosen due to morphine allergy or adverse effects such as nausea or itching. However, physicians must be aware that when selecting hydromorphone versus morphine there is a six fold difference in dosing, 0.1 mg/kg of morphine versus an equianalgesic dose of 0.015 mg/kg of hydromorphone which could contribute to dosing errors.

Nalbuphine is a commercially available μ-receptor agonist/antagonist and is used in some institutions for inpatient management of SCD pain. Woods et al (45) demonstrated nalbuphine to be as effective as intramuscular meperidine. A second retrospective study found patients treated with nalbuphine were less likely to develop acute chest syndrome and had a shorter hospital LOS than patients treated with morphine (46). No prospective trials have yet been published and at the moment, nalbuphine is not included in national SCD guidelines. It is more commonly used in the treatment of opioid-induced pruritis rather than a stand-alone analgesic.

Methadone, a synthetic analgesic with properties similar to morphine, has limited use in the treatment of inpatient acute painful episodes for children with SCD. Unlike morphine, it has an extremely long half-life that is estimated in adults to range from 19 to 36 hours (47). The true half-life of methadone in healthy children, much less children with SCD is unknown. The lack of information about methadone pharmacokinetics significantly limits adequate dosing intervals and treatment strategies based on established pharmacologic principles. Such a long half-life is impractical for the treatment of acute pain as steady state levels are not reached for five days, longer than the average LOS of 4.4 days for children with SCD pain (19). Furthermore, when methadone is used for the acute treatment of pain, dose escalation occurs frequently due to breakthrough pain which produces excessive sedation once steady-state has been reached, commonly four or five days after methadone initiation.

Codeine, is in general not appropriate for treating severe pain that has failed outpatient oral analgesics. It is most commonly used in its oral form to treat mild to moderate pain. Codeine doses over 65mg are not recommended as increases above this amount do not produce interval increases in analgesia, but still have increasing side effects (34). Codeine itself is not a μ-receptor agonist and must first be metabolized to the active drug, morphine, to produce pain relief. Genetic polymorphisms in the cytochrome p450 responsible for codeine metabolism, CYP2D6, exist and have been associated with poor analgesic efficacy in some populations. Lower CYP2D6 activity has been described in African-Americans(48) with 58% of children with SCD-Hb SS presenting to the ED in pain having reduced functioning alleles(49).

Meperidine is no longer recommended in the treatment of acute sickle cell pain in children or adults. Although meperidine may provide good analgesia and for many years was used as first line for sickle cell pain in the ED and inpatient unit, the potential toxicity of meperidine outweighs the clinical benefit. Meperidine toxicity primarily results from the production of normeperidine and its very different half-life from the active analgesic; three hours for meperidine versus 15 to 20 hours for normeperidine (50). As a result, if meperidine is given as a scheduled medication, normeperidine accumulates, causing neurotoxicity such as dysphoria, irritable mood, clonus and seizures. Meperidine toxicity occurs more commonly in patients with impaired renal function, though seizures have been reported in normal renal function (51) and with prolonged or repeated administration (50). The incidence of meperidine-induced seizures in children with SCD-Hb SS has been reported at 4 per 100 patients (52), an unacceptable risk benefit ratio in most settings.

Ketorolac is a newer non-opioid analgesic that has gained popularity in the treatment of sickle cell pain in some centers. Data supporting its use as a reasonable alternative to opioids is limited and inconsistent. A number of studies have evaluated the utility of ketorolac in the ED. Children who presented to the ED with severe pain and were given ketorolac demonstrated no difference in overall morphine use, pain intensity, rate of hospitalization, or ED return than children treated with morphine alone (53). Children with mild to moderate pain were able to be discharged after a single dose of ketorolac, but those with severe pain required additional opioids and admission (54). Ketorolac does not decrease overall opioid consumption (55). One study employing a continuous infusion of ketorolac, a method associated with increasing renal toxicity, did find patients needed fewer doses of intramuscular (IM) meperidine and had less pain than patients receiving as needed IM meperidine (56). The main toxicities associated with prolonged ketorolac use include renal failure and gastrointestinal bleeding. One case of irreversible renal failure after ketorolac administration in a child with sickle cell disease has been reported (57) and a second case of gastric perforation and death has occurred (58). Given the lack of documented benefit and the established toxicity, although perhaps rare, the use of ketorolac in the treatment of SCD pain is questionable.

Route of administration

Opioids are most commonly given IV in the ED or hospital for the treatment of acute sickle cell pain in children; adults more frequently receive IM therapy. Some research suggests that oral morphine can be as effective as IV morphine in treating pain (59). However, oral morphine was associated with an increased risk of developing acute chest syndrome (60). Transdermal, intranasal, and sublingual formulations of many opioid preparations exist but have not yet been evaluated systematically in patients with SCD and cannot be recommended as a treatment choice for acute management of pain.

Breakthrough pain

The recognition of breakthrough pain is necessary to improve pain management. Breakthrough pain is defined as an intense increase in pain that occurs with rapid onset even when pain control medication is being used (61). All inpatient orders for pain should include a strategy for the management of breakthrough pain. Perhaps the most efficient way to treat breakthrough pain is with a PCA given at a dose approximately 1/6 of the total amount of the hourly opioid infusion. When using a PCA, the lockout interval should be based on the pharmacokinetics of the opioid. For IV morphine administration, the PCA lockout period should be every 20 minutes, corresponding to the time of onset of the infusion; however, a shorter lockout period of 10 minutes would be inappropriate because morphine would not yet have reached peak analgesic effect and the patient could not be expected to have yet experienced pain relief. A 10 minute lockout is appropriate for IV fentanyl that has a shorter time of onset whereas hydromorphone has a longer time of onset and is best used with a 30 minute lockout.

If continuous medication is not being administered then the breakthrough pain dose should be approximately 1/3 to ¼ of the intermittent opioid dose (oral or IV). The biggest dilemma with this strategy is that nursing guidelines often allow as needed pain medications to be given within 60 minutes of the request. An hour delay from the onset of breakthrough pain to administration of analgesic is far too long for most patients. This may result in increased pain, increased requests for analgesics, development of behaviors consistent with pseudoaddiction and contribute to a less than optimal relationship between the patient, their perceived needs and nursing care.

PCA and continuous infusion titration

For patients placed on an opioid PCA with continuous infusion, it is appropriate to periodically adjust the basal or continuous opioid rate. As previously discussed, breatkthrough pain is best managed with PCA and clinician boluses. A patient who requires multiple additional doses, i.e. is receiving all allowable PCA doses each hour, should have their continuous infusion adjusted every six to eight hours. For example, a patient receives continuous morphine at 2 mg/hr. They self-administer and receive 3 PCA doses of 0.3 mg each in hour while receiving 2 additional clinician boluses of 1 mg of morphine. If we calculate the total amount of morphine the patient received, it is actually 2 mg/hr plus 2.9 mg/hr. Although the patient's orders read morphine 2 mg/hr, they actually received 4.9 mg/hr. Fear of respiratory depression often limits opioid titration. Given that the patient has already received this dose, respiratory depression should not be a worry. The clinician is only providing what they have already received.

Management of adverse effects of opioids

Opioid analgesics required to treat pain frequently produces unwanted adverse effects. The most common of these include itching, constipation, hallucinations and mood changes, but the most worrisome is respiratory depression. Many strategies exist to manage these effects though many have not been systematically evaluated in the literature.

Opioid induced pruritis (OIP) has previously been attributed to medication induced histamine release. More recent literature suggests pruritis is caused by activity at central μ-receptors rather than through histamine (62). Itching may occur after one dose or after multiple doses with any opioid medication and is more common with intrathecal administration. Because of the association with histamine release, antihistamines such as diphenhydramine are commonly employed in the treatment of OIP. Diphenhydramine, when given IV, can contribute to excessive sedation and should not routinely be used to treat OIP in SCD patients. In addition, diphenhydramine is ineffective in reducing OIP induced by morphine administration (62). Despite laboratory evidence, many practitioners find clinically that anti-histamines decrease symptoms. Cetirizine or other second generation anti-histamines cause less sedation and are more appropriate for patients with SCD. Research in the management of OIP now focuses on agents that are antagonists at the μ-receptor such as nalbuphine or naltrexone (63). Nalbuphine which is a mixed agonist/antagonist may be given as a continuous infusion along with the primary opioid analgesic. Doses should not exceed 2mg/hour to prevent decreased efficacy due to μ-receptor antagonism. Continuous naloxone has been used in the treatment of OIP in adults but has not been systematically evaluated in children. Severe itching, hallucinations and mood changes may best be managed with opioid rotation (64), for instance changing from morphine to hydromorphone or from hydromorphone to fentanyl if adverse effects persist (see table 3).

Constipation is the most common side effects of opioid administration. Prophylactic therapy for prevention of constipation should be standard for any child admitted for management of pain. No evidence based guidelines have been published describing the most effective strategy to prevent constipation among children admitted to the hospital for pain with sickle cell disease. Therapy for prevention of constipation can be divided into three main categories: bulk agents (psyllium), osmotic agents (lactulose or polyethylene glycol), and stimulants (bisacodyl or sennasoids). Osmotic or bulk agents alone are insufficient to prevent constipation. Patients should be treated with a stimulant to overcome opioid-induced ileus(34) (see table 4).

Table 3. Management of opioid-induced pruritis

Medication	Dose	Recommendation
Antihistamines Diphenhydramine Cetirizine	 1 mg/kg po q 6 hrs prn itching 6-12 months 2.5 mg daily 12-23 months 2.5 mg BID 2-5 years 5mg daily ≥ 5 years 5mg BID	May be clinically effective, but evidence lacking. Not recommended due to sedation. Any second generation anti-histamine may be used first line (i.e. hydroxyzine or loratadine).
Nalbuphine Intermittent Dosing Continuous Infusion	 0.03-0.05mg/kg/dose q1 hr prn itching 0.025mg/kg/hr, max dose 2mg/hr	Preferred method and supported by current evidence. Higher doses can antagonize analgesic effect.
Naloxone		Not well studied for pruritis in children.

Table 4. Prevention of opioid-induced constipation

Medication	Dosing	Recommendation
Bulk Agents	i.e. fiber	Not recommended.
Stool Softeners	i.e. colace	Not recommended.
Stimulants Senna Bisacodyl (Tablets only)	 1 mo-2 yrs 1.25 ml daily *(2.2 mg sennosides; max dose 8.8 mg/day)* 2 - <6 yrs 2.5 ml daily *(4.4 mg sennosides; max dose 8.8 mg/day)* 6 - 12 yrs 1 tablet daily *(8.8 mg sennosides; max dose 17.6 mg/day)* >12 yrs 2 tablets daily *(17.6 mg sennosides; max dose 35.2 mg/day)* < 3yrs 5-10 mg po daily 3-12 yrs 5-10 mg po/pr daily >12 yrs 5-15 mg po/pr daily	Preferred Method.
Osmotic Agents Lactulose Polyethylene Glycol (MiraLax)	 > 6 mo (10gm/15 ml) 1-2 ml/kg divided BID to TID Adults - 17 gm in 8 oz of liquid daily to BID Children (MiraLax soln) 10 kg – 2 oz daily to BID 20 kg - 4 oz daily to BID 30 kg - 5 oz daily to BID 40 kg – 7 oz daily to BID 50 + kg – Adult dosing	May be used in combination with stimulant.

Supportive measures

The prompt treatment of dehydration is an important for any patient, including those with sickle cell disease that present with pain. However, there is no evidence that intravenous hydration will hasten recovery to baseline in children with sickle cell disease and pain. A recent Cochrane database publication found no studies that could be used to evaluate the efficacy of IV fluids in acute SCD pain (65). Use of IVF boluses in the emergency department during initial presentation for acute pain did not increase the likelihood of ED discharge (66,67). Some data exist suggesting excessive hydration may be harmful leading to pulmonary edema (68). Rapid infusion of isotonic fluids should be reserved for children with hypovolemia. Otherwise, total fluid administration (oral and IV) should not exceed 1500 to 2000 ml/m2/day.

Previous research has established a link between acute pain episodes and the acute chest syndrome. The use of incentive spirometry decreased the rate of acute chest syndrome in a randomized trial and, although it does not treat pain itself, has become standard care in patients experiencing a VOE (69). Oxygen for the treatment of oxygen desaturation is appropriate; however, equally important is an evaluation as to why oxygen saturation dropped. Prophylactic oxygen has not been shown to decrease duration of hospital stay or pain intensity (38) and may mask acute changes in respiratory status when the earliest sign would be a drop in oxygen saturation.

Simple transfusion is not recommended in the treatment of acute sickle cell pain (9). It may play a role in decreasing frequency of painful episodes when applied as a program of chronic transfusion but has not been shown to alter the natural history of an active acute episode. Steroids may be used to treat asthma and acute respiratory conditions that occur concomitantly with painful episodes. Steroids chiefly for pain have not been investigated and should be approached with caution.

Recent publications suggest a higher readmission rate in patients who received steroids for acute chest syndrome (70) and an increased rate of acute cerebral hemorrhage when combined with antecedent blood transfusion (71).

Adjuvant therapies for the treatment of pain such as heating pads, whirlpool therapy, and massage may improve pain relief. Behavioral therapies such as distraction techniques, play therapy and coping techniques are important in both the inpatient and outpatient treatment of SCD pain. Multi-modal therapy incorporating child life therapists, social workers, psychologists, occupational and physical therapists should be used to maximize pain relief.

Weaning intravenous pain medication

In many teaching hospitals, inpatient management of SCD pain may result in contact with as many as eight physicians (day and nighttime house staff team) and three nurses (eight-hour shifts) within a 24 hour period. Thus, clear and simple guidelines are important to insure pain relief. There are no evidence based guidelines for the optimal strategy of treatment of pain; however, we employ a strategy for pain management that has been satisfactory to most patients and decreases the variability in treatment philosophy from one physician to another.

Based on our practice, a simple and user-friendly approach for both the patient and physician, in the first 24 hours following admission, no weaning of pain medication is done unless evidence of excessive opioid administration exists. If the patient does not awaken in severe pain overnight, we elect to decrease the pain medication by 20% prior to 0600 the following morning.

This approach allows for the family and the patient to understand the plan before being implemented. In addition the house staff or attending assigned to evaluate the patient in the morning has at least a six hour window to discuss whether the 20% decrease in pain medication dose provides inadequate pain relief. No further weaning is done for the remainder of the day, and evening signout discourages further weaning, unless there is evidence of excessive opioid administration.

The same weaning method is followed for the subsequent morning with a decrease of 20% of the original dose. This practice is repeated until the patient has an IV dose that is either equivalent or close to the patients maintenance pain plan for home (see figure 3).

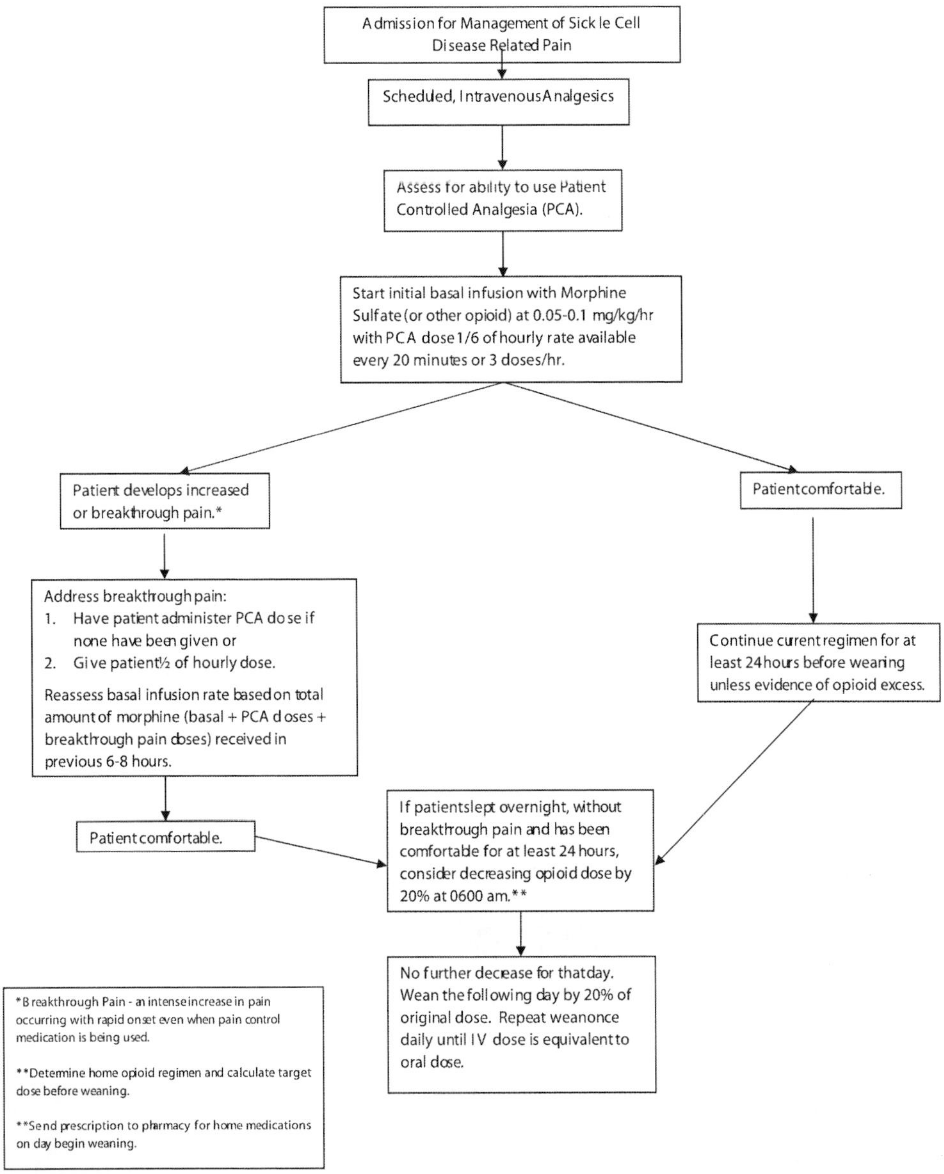

Figure 3. Flow diagram for the treatment of children with sickle cell disease admitted for pain.

Preparing for discharge

As patients reach phases 6 and 7, pain begins to resolve and IV medications should be gradually weaned. The inappropriate conversion of patients receiving high doses of intravenous opioids to lower doses oral analgesics can precipitate withdrawal symptoms, increase pain intensity and put patients at risk for hospital readmission (72). It should not be expected that pain will be completely resolved at discharge but the patient, caregiver and healthcare should perceived adequate pain control on oral analgesics prior to discharge. In addition, pain medications should be scheduled for 48-72 hours after discharge and should be given to the patient prior to discharge rather than a prescription to be filled elsewhere. Follow-up should be scheduled within 7-14 days of discharge especially in children with co-morbid asthma, steroid administration, or frequent pain episodes. Children with SCD should receive follow-up care by a hematologist or physician with expertise in SCD. Children followed by a specialist have fewer hospitalizations and ED visits than those not followed by a specialty clinic(73) (see appendix 2).

Conclusions

SCD pain is the most challenging condition for patients to experience and physicians to treat successfully. We have identified ten actions that can be taken by healthcare providers to improve the treatment of sickle cell pain in children (see table 5). The most important is to believe the child is in pain. Other simple behaviors include scheduling intravenous pain medications, delaying dose decreases once the child is comfortable until after the first 24 hours, using alternative strategies while in the hospital such as child life, decreasing doses in the morning when caregivers and physicians are available, decreasing the dose daily by 20% until reaching an appropriate dose for oral conversion, giving the patient discharge medications instead of discharge prescriptions, scheduling oral analgesics at home, preparing a pain action plan, and providing the patient with the date and time of follow-up with a physician experienced in the care of SCD.

The appropriate management of acute pain in children with SCD involves the active participation of patients, parents, nurses, physicians, social workers, child life personal, and psychologists. Care should be multi-dimensional involving pharmacologic methods as well as behavioral, psychological and physical interventions. Education and consistency in medication administration is essential in enabling families to manage pain at home and to recognize when higher-level of care is needed.

Table 5. Ten key actions in the successful management of sickle cell disease related pain in children

1. Believe the child is in pain.
2. Schedule opioid pain medications. *As needed or PRN orders are not acceptable for children in pain.
3. If the child is comfortable, don't wean for the first 24 hours of hospitalization.
4. Wean in the morning when caregivers, physicians and primary nurses are available to assess results.
5. Wean by 20% daily until reaching an appropriate dose to convert to oral analgesics.
6. Use non-traditional strategies for pain management, i.e. child life therapists, psychologists, or physical and occupational therapists.
7. Give the patient discharge medications, not a prescription to be filled.
8. Schedule oral pain medications for 48 to 72 hours at home after discharge.
9. Develop a pain action plan and educate the patient and caregivers on how to use it.
10. Schedule a follow-up appointment with the patient's hematologist within 7-14 days after discharge.

Appendix I

Children's
HOSPITAL • ST. LOUIS

HEMATOLOGY / ONCOLOGY ORDERS FOR MORPHINE PCA & INFUSIONS

ALL ORDERS MUST HAVE DATE, TIME WRITTEN, WRITER'S AND TRANSCRIBER'S LEGIBLE SIGNATURE (FIRST INITIAL, LAST NAME, TITLE) AND TRANSCRIPTION TIME. DIAGNOSIS AND ALLERGIES TO BE INCLUDED IN ALL ADMIT ORDERS.

Attending: **Unit:**

Diagnosis:

Allergies: (List or note NKA) **Height:** **Weight:**

Authorization is hereby given to dispense the generic or chemical equivalent unless otherwise indicated by the words "No Substitute."

Date	Time Written	Orders – Signatures – Transcription Times
		1. No orders for opioid analgesics or sedative medications shall be transcribed or given to this patient while on PCA/continuous IV opioid infusion unless authorized by attending physician or unit supervising resident.
		2. Post sign at bedside: Only patient to push PCA button.
		3. For respiratory rate less than ________ call house officer and stop PCA.
		4. Assess and record developmentally appropriate pain score every 2 hours while awake (choose one developmentally appropriate scale).
		5. Assess and record sedation level every 2 hours.
		6. Continuous monitoring with pulse oximeter, record saturation every hour (mandatory for all patients on continuous opioid infusions).
		7. Call house officer for O_2 saturation less than ________% and place 100% O_2 per face mask on patient.
		Drug: Morphine **Concentration: 1 mg/ml**
		CONTINUOUS MORPHINE INFUSION PLUS PCA - WITH HEME/ONC ATTENDING APPROVAL ONLY (DOCUMENT IN CHART)
		☐ Yes ☐ No 8. Continuous opioid infusion via Computorized PCA pump Normal starting dose for sickle cell disease patients (0.05 - 0.1 mg/kg/hr) *Recommended max starting dose is 4 mg/hr.* Normal starting dose for oncology patients (0.03 - 0.05 mg/kg/hr) Initial infusion rate: ________mg/kg/hr = ________ mg/hr = ________ ml/hr
		☐ Yes ☐ No 9. Computerized PCA pump — Typical range PCA dose:________mg — 0.17 x continuous infusion rate (mg/hr) ☐ Yes ☐ No Lockout Time:______minutes — (20 minutes) ☐ Yes ☐ No One hour limit:______(max. number of doses) — (3) ☐ Yes ☐ No Clinician Bolus:________(specify dose) 0.17 x continuous infusion rate (mg/hr) every _____ minutes prn unrelieved pain
		Signature ________ Printed Name ________ Date / Time ________

DO NOT WRITE IN BARCODE AREA

CN 3-7400-420 EF (06/25/07) Page 1 of 2

CN 3-7400-420 EF

White: Chart
Canary: Pharmacy

TAB: ORDER SHEET

Appendix I. (Continued)

Children's
HOSPITAL • ST. LOUIS
BJC HealthCare

HEMATOLOGY / ONCOLOGY ORDERS FOR MORPHINE PCA & INFUSIONS

ALL ORDERS MUST HAVE DATE, TIME WRITTEN, WRITER'S AND TRANSCRIBER'S LEGIBLE SIGNATURE (FIRST INITIAL, LAST NAME, TITLE) AND TRANSCRIPTION TIME. DIAGNOSIS AND ALLERGIES TO BE INCLUDED IN ALL ADMIT ORDERS.

Attending: **Unit:**

Diagnosis:

Allergies: (List or note NKA) **Height:** **Weight:**

Authorization is hereby given to dispense the generic or chemical equivalent unless otherwise indicated by the words "No Substitute."

Date	Time Written	Orders – Signatures – Transcription Times
		1. No orders for opioid analgesics or sedative medications shall be transcribed or given to this patient while on PCA/continuous IV opioid infusion unless authorized by attending physician or unit supervising resident.
		2. Post sign at bedside: Only patient to push PCA button.
		3. For respiratory rate less than ________ call house officer and stop PCA.
		4. Assess and record developmentally appropriate pain score every 2 hours while awake (choose one developmentally appropriate scale).
		5. Assess and record sedation level every 2 hours.
		6. Continuous monitoring with pulse oximeter, record saturation every hour (mandatory for all patients on continuous opioid infusions).
		7. Call house officer for O_2 saturation less than ________% and place 100% O_2 per face mask on patient.
		Drug: Morphine **Concentration: 1 mg/ml**
		CONTINUOUS MORPHINE INFUSION PLUS PCA - WITH HEME/ONC ATTENDING APPROVAL ONLY (DOCUMENT IN CHART)
		☐ Yes ☐ No 8. Continuous opioid infusion via Computerized PCA pump Normal starting dose for sickle cell disease patients (0.05 - 0.1 mg/kg/hr) *Recommended max starting dose is 4 mg/hr.* Normal starting dose for oncology patients (0.03 - 0.05 mg/kg/hr) Initial infusion rate: ________mg/kg/hr = ________ mg/hr = ________ ml/hr
		☐ Yes ☐ No 9. Computerized PCA pump — Typical range PCA dose:________mg — 0.17 x continuous infusion rate (mg/hr) ☐ Yes ☐ No Lockout Time:________minutes — (20 minutes) ☐ Yes ☐ No One hour limit:________(max. number of doses) — (3) ☐ Yes ☐ No Clinician Bolus:________(specify dose) 0.17 x continuous infusion rate (mg/hr) every ______ minutes prn unrelieved pain
		Signature ________ Printed Name ________ Date / Time ________

DO NOT WRITE IN BARCODE AREA

CN 3-7400-420 EF (06/25/07) Page 1 of 2

White: Chart
Canary: Pharmacy

TAB: ORDER SHEET

CN 3-7400-420 EF

Children's
HOSPITAL · ST. LOUIS
HealthCare

HEMATOLOGY / ONCOLOGY ORDERS FOR MORPHINE PCA & INFUSIONS

ALL ORDERS MUST HAVE DATE, TIME WRITTEN, WRITER'S AND TRANSCRIBER'S LEGIBLE SIGNATURE (FIRST INITIAL, LAST NAME, TITLE) AND TRANSCRIPTION TIME. DIAGNOSIS AND ALLERGIES TO BE INCLUDED IN ALL ADMIT ORDERS.

Attending: **Unit:**

Diagnosis:

Allergies: (List or note NKA) **Height:** **Weight:**

Authorization is hereby given to dispense the generic or chemical equivalent unless otherwise indicated by the words "No Substitute."

Date	Time Written	Orders – Signatures – Transcription Times
		☐ Yes ☐ No 10. Senna ☐ 1 month - 2 years: 1.25 ml syrup po every hs (2.2 mg sennosides). Max dose 8.8 mg/day. ☐ 2 - <6 years: 2.5 ml syrup po every hs (4.4 mg sennosides). Max dose 8.8 mg/day. ☐ 6 - 12 years: 1 tablet po every hs (8.8 mg sennosides). Max dose 17.2 mg/day. ☐ >12 years: 2 tablets po every hs (17.6 mg sennosides). Max dose 34.4 mg/day
		☐ Yes ☐ No 11. For pruritus: (*Avoid IV benadryl due to sedative effects.*) Cetirizine ☐ 6 - 12 mo: 2.5 mg po once a day prn pruritus. ☐ 12 - 23 mo: 2.5 mg po every 12 hrs prn pruritus. ☐ 2- 5 years: 5 mg po once a day or may be divided every 12 hrs prn pruritus. ☐ ≥6 years: 5 mg po every 12 hrs prn pruritus. *For itching not relieved by Cetirizine, consider Nalbuphine.*
		☐ Yes ☐ No 12. Nalbuphine 0.03 - 0.05 mg/kg/dose = ________mg IV every 1 hr prn pruritus. Max dose 2mg. If pruritus not relieved after 2 hrs, consider nalbuphine 0.025 mg/kg/hr continuous drip (max 2 mg/hr).
		13. Naloxone 10 mcg/kg = ________mcg (max dose 1000 mcg) IV prn respiratory depression available on floor while patient receiving continuous infusion.
		14. MD to assess PCA doses every 12 hrs and adjust maintenance dose appropriately.
		Signature / Printed Name / Date / Time

DO NOT WRITE IN BARCODE AREA

CN 3-7400-420 EF (06/25/07) Page 2 of 2

White: Chart
Canary: Pharmacy

TAB: ORDER SHEET

CN 3-7400-420 EF

Appendix I. (Continued)

Children's
HOSPITAL • ST. LOUIS

HEMATOLOGY / ONCOLOGY ORDERS FOR MORPHINE PCA & INFUSIONS

ALL ORDERS MUST HAVE DATE, TIME WRITTEN, WRITER'S AND TRANSCRIBER'S LEGIBLE SIGNATURE (FIRST INITIAL, LAST NAME, TITLE) AND TRANSCRIPTION TIME. DIAGNOSIS AND ALLERGIES TO BE INCLUDED IN ALL ADMIT ORDERS.

Attending: **Unit:**

Diagnosis:

Allergies: (List or note NKA) **Height:** **Weight:**

Authorization is hereby given to dispense the generic or chemical equivalent unless otherwise indicated by the words "No Substitute."

Date	Time Written	Orders – Signatures – Transcription Times
		☐ Yes ☐ No 10. Senna ☐ 1 month - 2 years: 1.25 ml syrup po every hs (2.2 mg sennosides). Max dose 8.8 mg/day. ☐ 2 - <6 years: 2.5 ml syrup po every hs (4.4 mg sennosides). Max dose 8.8 mg/day. ☐ 6- 12 years: 1 tablet po every hs (8.8 mg sennosides). Max dose 17.2 mg/day. ☐ >12 years: 2 tablets po every hs (17.6 mg sennosides). Max dose 34.4 mg/day
		☐ Yes ☐ No 11. For pruritus: (*Avoid IV benadryl due to sedative effects.*) Cetirizine ☐ 6 - 12 mo: 2.5 mg po once a day prn pruritus. ☐ 12 - 23 mo: 2.5 mg po every 12 hrs prn pruritus. ☐ 2- 5 years: 5 mg po once a day or may be divided every 12 hrs prn pruritus. ☐ ≥6 years: 5 mg po every 12 hrs prn pruritus. *For itching not relieved by Cetirizine, consider Nalbuphine.*
		☐ Yes ☐ No 12. Nalbuphine 0.03 - 0.05 mg/kg/dose = ________mg IV every 1 hr prn pruritus. Max dose 2mg. If pruritus not relieved after 2 hrs, consider nalbuphine 0.025 mg/kg/hr continuous drip (max 2 mg/hr).
		13. Naloxone 10 mcg/kg = _________mcg (max dose 1000 mcg) IV prn respiratory depression available on floor while patient receiving continuous infusion.
		14. MD to assess PCA doses every 12 hrs and adjust maintenance dose appropriately.
		Signature / Printed Name / Date / Time

DO NOT WRITE IN BARCODE AREA

CN 3-7400-420 EF (06/25/07) Page 2 of 2

CN 3-7400-420 EF

White: Chart
Canary: Pharmacy

TAB: ORDER SHEET

Appendix II

Children's
HOSPITAL • ST. LOUIS
BJC HealthCare

VASO-OCCLUSIVE EPISODE DISCHARGE ORDERS

Primary Care Provider: ____________________ (NAME) ____________ (PHONE) Attending Physician: ____________________ (NAME) ____________ (PHONE)

Active Diagnoses:	Chronic Asthma Severity:	Established Diagnoses:
1. Vaso-occlusive episode 2. ____________ 3. ____________	☐ Mild Intermittent ☐ Moderate Persistent ☐ Mild Persistent ☐ Severe Persistant	1. ____________ 2. ____________ 3. ____________

Hospital Course / Procedures / Consults

☐ Received IV pain medication: ____________. Was weaned over the course of ___ days. Started on oral medications on hospital day ___. Pain was controlled on oral analgesics as assessed by the patient/caregiver at discharge.
☐ Received steroids, Atrovent, and frequent albuterol. Breathing comfortably and tolerating albuterol every 4 hours by discharge.
☐ Received oxygen for hypoxia. Saturations at baseline and off supplemental oxygen for ≥ 24 hours at discharge.
☐ Received ____________ *(type)* blood transfusion for: ____________
☐ Other: ____________

Complete List of Medications (Name)	Dose	How to Give	How Often to Give / Time
☐ ____________ *(Long-acting opioid)*		By Mouth	Every 12 hours for 2 days, then as needed following Pain Action Plan
☐ ____________ *(Short-acting opioid)*		By Mouth	Every 4 hours as needed for breakthrough pain.
☐ Folic Acid	1mg (1 tablet)	By Mouth	Everyday
☐ Penicillin	☐ 125 mg ________ ☐ 250 mg ________	By Mouth	Twice a day, every day.
☐ Albuterol	☐ 2 puffs ☐ ____________	Inhaler with spacer In nebulizer	Every 4 hours for 2 days, then every 6 hours for 1 week, then as needed following Asthma Action Plan
☐ Oral Steroid: ☐ Prednisone ☐ Orapred (Prednisolone)	______mg (___ tablet(s)) ______mg (______ ml)	By Mouth	Every morning for _____ days. ☐ Extra dose(s) for future use following action plan.
☐ ____________ *(inhaled steroid/strength)*			
☐ ____________ *(Leukotriene Modifier/strength)*			
☐ ____________ *(home nocturnal oxygen)*			
☐ ____________			
☐ ____________			

☐ Staff to send re-labeled medications home with patient
☐ Medication list continues on separate page ☐ Home Medications ☐ No previous Home Medications

Follow-Up Appointments / Tests	Date / Time	Location	Phone	Fax
☐ ____________ *(SCD Team within one week)*				

Instructions

1. Discharge: ☐ Home ☐ Other: ____________
2. Follow Pain Action Plan. Discussed and copies given.
3. Bring all discharge papers, medications and equipment to follow-up appointments.
4. May return to school/daycare/usual activities within 2 days. No gym, outdoor play or strenuous activity for 1 week. Note given for school.
5. Diet: ☐ Resume usual diet ☐ Other: ____________
6. Other: ____________

I understand this information and am able to follow the above instructions.

Signature of Patient / Parent / Legal guardian	Relationship	Date / Time
Signature of Discharging RN	Printed Name of Discharging RN	Date / Time
Signature of Physician / APN	Printed Name of Physician / APN	Date / Time

Discharge Summary to be dictated by: ____________ Attending of Record: ____________

It is the responsibility of the discharging physician to ensure all unsigned verbal orders are authenticated prior to discharge of the patient.
Reviewed by: ____________

DO NOT WRITE IN BARCODE AREA CN 7-7400-1041 EF (10/24/07)

CN 7-7400-1041 EF

TAB: ORDERS

Appendix III

Types and Characteristics of Pain Associated With Sickle Cell Disease

Acute Pain

- Characterized by an episodic, abrupt, and unpredictable onset of pain for which there is no other explanation

Types of Pain

- Acute painful event
  - sudden onset
  - pain in any and all parts of the body
- Acute hand-foot syndrome
  - painful swelling of the back of hands and feet
  - may affect only one hand or foot
  - maybe confused with osteomyelitis
- Acute Chest Syndrome
  - chest pain particularly rib and substernal
  - may be associated with fever, fast breathing, and/or hypoxia
- Splenic Sequestration
  - pain in the upper left quadrant
  - paleness and weakness often occurs and should be considered medical emergency
  - treatment includes blood transfusion, parent education, and possibly splenectomy
- Hepatic sequestration
  - pain in the upper right quadrant
  - sudden decreased in hemoglobin
  - enlarged liver
- Abdominal Pain
  - jaundice (yellow color eyes)
  - pain in the upper right part of the abdomen associated with gall bladder disease (cholelithiasis) particularly when eating fatting foods
- Priapism (painful erection of penis)
  - may last for a few hours to day or may be chronic or intermittent
- Avascular necrosis of femur or humerus
  - prolonged constant bone pain in knee, hip or shoulder

Summary of Phases of the Chronology of Pain in Children and Adolescents with Sickle Cell Disease

Phase I – Baseline
Phase II - Pre-Pain
Phase III - Pain Start Point
Phase IV - Pain Acceleration
Phase V - Peak Pain Experience
Phase VI - Pain Decrease Start Point
Phase VII - Steady Pain Decline
Phase VIII - Pain Resolution

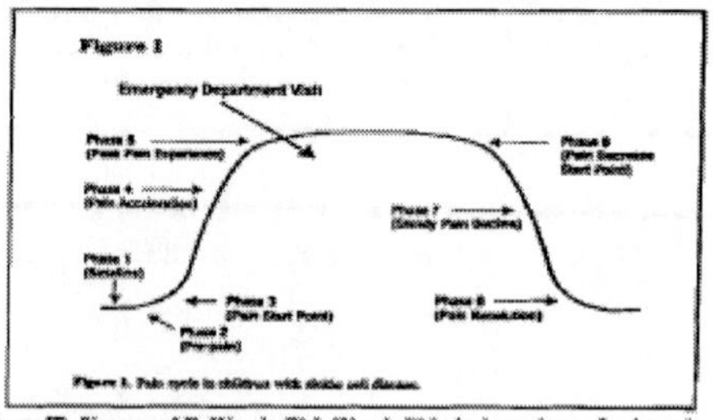

Beyer JE. Simmons LE. Woods GM. Woods PM. A chronology of pain and comfort in children with sickle cell disease. Archives of Pediatrics & Adolescent Medicine. 153(9):913-20, 1999 Sep. 99409931

Phase 2 Pre-Pain Phase

- Your child may show no evidence of pain but many begin to display some signs and symptoms of a painful episode.
- Caregivers acknowledged that they were able to see the episode of pain coming before the pain actually begins, for instance your child may have jaundiced (yellow) eyes.
- Mild pain medications, such as acetaminophen or ibuprofen are initiated.

Phase 3 Pain Start

- Pain starts off as mild usually located in one specific area.
- Pain medications, such as MSIR, OxyContin, or Tylenol with codeine.

Phase 4 Pain Acceleration

- Stronger pain medications (Tylenol with codeine, MSIR, or OxyIR).
- Typically your child will not attend school during this time period.
- Non medicinal pain measures may be helpful (sleep, radio, homework, television).

Phase 5 Peak Pain Experience

- Your child may be unable to relieve their own pain and must come to the hospital.
- Your child may describe their pain as: stabbing, drilling, pounding, banging or throbbing.
- Your child's pain may not decrease until 2 or 3 days later.

Phase 6 Pain Decrease Start Point

- Your child starts to feel better and may start to do other activities like attend school in the hospital, and play games.

Phase 7 Steady Pain Decline

- Your child will begin to show improvement and will have better mobility and improved appetite.
- Your child will be usually discharged from the hospital on OxyContin or OxyIR.

Phase 8 Pain Resolution

- Children resume normal behavior, appearance, and mood.

Medical Treatment of Pain in Children and Adolescents with Sickle Cell Disease
(HgbSS, HgbSC, Hgbβ°, HbgSβ⁺)

Medical Record #____________________

Name: ____________________ Primary Nurse/Practitioner: ____________________

DOB: ____________________ Primary Hematologist: ____________________

Date: ____________________ Weight: ____________________

Phase 2

1. Acetaminophen____________ or
   Ibuprofen ____________ every 4 to 6 hours for 24 hours.
2. If pain increases or continues then go to medical treatment for phase 3.

Choose one of three options A, B, or C

Phase 3 – Option A

1. Morphine Sulfate Immediate Release (MSIR) ______________.
2. MSIR - if no relief from MSIR in one hour, repeat same dose.
3. If there is improvement from MSIR, start MS Contin ____________ 1 hour after the last dose of MSIR.

Phase 3 – Option B

1. OxyContin ______________.
2. If no improvement in 1 hour call 454-6000 ask for the hematologist on call.
3. If pain is controlled for more than two hours but additional pain occurs, take OxyIR ________,

Phase 3 – Option C

1. Tylenol with codeine ______________.
2. If no improvement in 1 hour, start option A or option B.

Appendix III. (Continued)

Medical Treatment of Pain in Children and Adolescents with Sickle Cell Disease
(HgbSS, HgbSC, Hgbß °, HbgSß+)

Phase 4 -Option A and Option B

1. If there is pain becomes **worse** after the **first** MSIR **(Plan A)** Call (314) 454-6000 and ask for the hematologist on call.
2. If there is **no** improvement after the **second** MSIR in 1 hour call **(Plan A)** (314) 454-6000 and ask for hematologist on call.
3. If there is **no** improvement after **two hours** of OxyContin call **(Plan B)** (314) 454-6000 and ask for the hematologist on call.

You will be referred to the Hematology Clinic if before 12 P.M. or Emergency Department if after 12 P.M.

Phase 5- Peak Pain Experience

1. In the Emergency Department, 0.1mg/kg-0.15mg/kg morphine IV every 15 minutes until pain is controlled. If no relief in 2 hours or 0.2 mg/kg given, you will be admitted to the hospital.

Date:____________________

Patient Name____________________ Medical Record# ____________

Please circle size/amount tablets to be taken:

Medication	Quantity	Time Taken
OxyFast (Roxicodone) - 20mg/1cc	________	________
OxyIR (Roxicodone)- 5mg tablets	________	________
OxyContin - 10mg, 20mg, 40mg,	________	________
80mg, and 160mg tablets	________	________
MS Contin - 30mg, 60mg or 100mg tablets	________	________
MSIR- 15mg or 30mg tablets	________	________
Codeine (30mg) with Acetaminophen (325mg) is equal to Tylenol #3		________
Codeine (60mg) with Acetaminophen (325mg) is equal to Tylenol #4		________
Oxycodone (5 mg) with Acetaminophen (325mg) is equal to Percocet tablet.		________
Oxycodone (5 mg) with Acetaminophen (500mg) is equal to Percocet capsule.		________

Wong-Baker Faces Pain Rating Scale

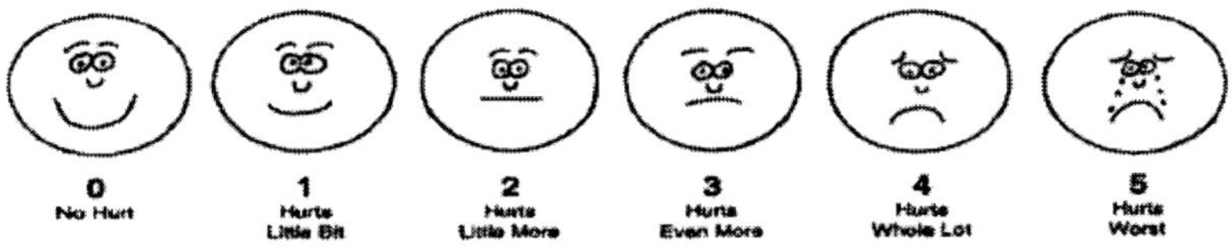

0–10 Numeric Pain Intensity Scale

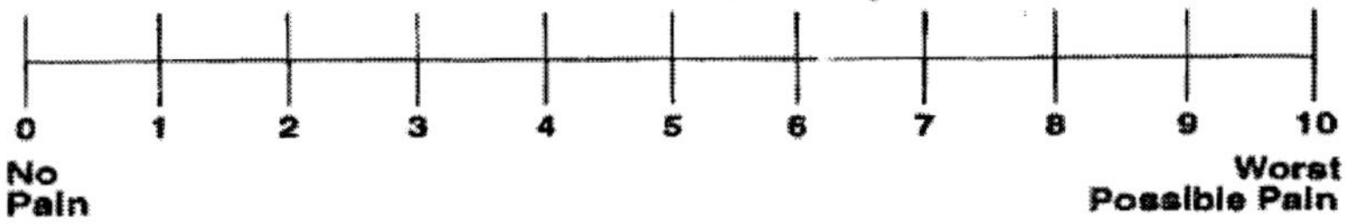

Appendix IV

Staple

Children's
HOSPITAL • ST. LOUIS
BJC HealthCare

ADMISSION ORDERS
VASO-OCCLUSIVE EPISODE
INTERMITTENT DOSE OPIOID
Recommended Age <7 years

ALL ORDERS MUST HAVE DATE, TIME WRITTEN, WRITER'S AND TRANSCRIBER'S LEGIBLE SIGNATURE (FIRST INITIAL, LAST NAME, TITLE) AND TRANSCRIPTION TIME. DIAGNOSIS AND ALLERGIES TO BE INCLUDED IN ALL ADMIT ORDERS.

Attending: **Unit:**

Diagnosis: Hgb S ___
Vaso-occlusive Episode
☐Y ☐N Asthma (Complete Asthma Section)
Other:

Allergies: (List or note NKA) **Height:** **Weight:**

Authorization is hereby given to dispense the generic or chemical equivalent unless otherwise indicated by the words "No Substitute."

Date	Time Written	Orders – Signatures – Transcription Times
		Condition:
		Nursing/Vitals: Temp, HR and RR every ______ (2-4 hrs), BP every 4 hrs, Oxygen Saturations every 4 hrs. Continuous pulse oximetry. Notify HO for: HR > ______, RR > ______ or < ______, Temp ≥ 38.5°C, no UOP in > 8 hrs, worsening pain, sats ≤ 92% RA, or an increasing oxygen requirement.
		Respiratory: FiO_2 to keep sats ≥ 92%. Wean to room air for sats ≥ 92%. Incentive Spirometry: 10 breaths/hr while awake and recorded by nurse. ☐ Yes ☐ No Home nocturnal oxygen: ______________________ (if yes, amount).
		Diet:
		IV Fluids: D5½ NS with 20 meq KCL/L at ________ ml/hr. IVF + PO to equal 1500 to 2000 ml/m2/day. Reassess IVF needs every 24 hrs. May heplock IV and discontinue fluids if taking adequate po fluids.
		Activity: As tolerated. After 24 hours, begin ambulation for 10 minutes every 8 hrs.
		Laboratory: On Admission: CBC w/ diff, reticulocyte count if not done in ED or clinic. CBC w/ diff, reticulocyte count every day. BUN and creatinine on hospital day 1 for patients age 12 or older. ☐ Yes ☐ No Type and screen if hemoglobin ≥ 1 gm/dl below baseline. ☐ Yes ☐ No ALT, AST, fractionated bilirubin if concern for increased icterus.
		Signature ______ Printed Name ______ Date / Time ______

DO NOT WRITE IN BARCODE AREA

CN 6-7400-950 EF (06/20/07) Page 1 of 5

CN 6-7400-950

TAB: ORDERS

Children's
HOSPITAL • ST. LOUIS
BJC HealthCare

ADMISSION ORDERS
VASO-OCCLUSIVE EPISODE
INTERMITTENT DOSE OPIOID
Recommended Age <7 years

ALL ORDERS MUST HAVE DATE, TIME WRITTEN, WRITER'S AND TRANSCRIBER'S LEGIBLE SIGNATURE (FIRST INITIAL, LAST NAME, TITLE) AND TRANSCRIPTION TIME. DIAGNOSIS AND ALLERGIES TO BE INCLUDED IN ALL ADMIT ORDERS.

Attending: **Unit:**

Diagnosis:

Allergies: (List or note NKA) **Height:** **Weight:**

Authorization is hereby given to dispense the generic or chemical equivalent unless otherwise indicated by the words "No Substitute."

Date	Time Written	Orders – Signatures – Transcription Times
		Pain Medications: Analgesics should be scheduled for all acute pain episodes. ☐ Yes ☐ No **MORPHINE SULFATE** 1. Morphine Sulfate (0.1 mg/kg/max dose 5 mg) = ________ mg IV every 2 hrs. **If patient is comfortable, do not wean dose for first 24 hours, except for adverse effects such as excessive sedation or respiratory depression.* ***If patient remains uncomfortable 20 minutes after current dose, then give Morphine Sulfate 0.05 mg/kg IV every 30 minutes until comfortable. (Max dose 0.3 mg/kg or 6 doses.) If unable to produce adequate analgesia, consider starting a continuous infusion or an alternative opioid.* 2. Breakthrough Pain: Morphine Sulfate ________ mg IV ($\frac{1}{3}$ to $\frac{1}{4}$ of scheduled dose as needed for increased pain every 30 minutes. Notify HO if patient requires > 2 doses. ☐ Yes ☐ No **HYDROMORPHONE - Not recommended for patients ≤ 20 kg.** 3. Hydromorphone (0.015 mg/kg/max dose 1 mg) = ________ mg IV every 3 hrs. **If patient is comfortable, do not wean dose for first 24 hours, except for adverse effects such as excessive sedation or respiratory depression.* ***If patient remains uncomfortable 30 minutes after current dose, then give Hydromorphone 0.008 mg/kg IV every 1 hour until comfortable. (Max 3 doses). If unable to produce adequate analgesia, consider starting a continuous infusion.* 4. Breakthrough Pain: Hydromorphone ______ mg IV ($\frac{1}{3}$ to $\frac{1}{4}$ of scheduled dose as needed for increased pain every 30 minutes. Notify HO if patient requires > 2 doses.
		Adjuvant Pain Medications: ☐ Yes ☐ No 1. Ibuprofen 10 mg/kg = ________ mg po every 6 hrs unless contraindicated. ** If patient unable to tolerate ibuprofen, consider acetaminophen at 15 mg/kg po every 6 hrs scheduled. Toradol po or IV not recommended.* 2. For pruritus: *(Avoid IV benadryl due to sedative effects.)* ☐ Yes ☐ No a. Cetirizine ☐ 6-12 mo 2.5 mg po every day prn pruritus ☐ 12-23 mo 2.5 mg po every 12 hrs prn pruritus ☐ 2-5 yrs 5 mg po every day or may be divided every 12 hrs prn pruritus ☐ ≥ 6 yrs 5 mg po every 12 hrs prn pruritus *For itching not relieved by Cetirizine, consider Nalbuphine.* ☐ Yes ☐ No b. Nalbuphine 0.03-0.05 mg/kg/dose = _______ mg (max dose 2 mg) IV every 1 hr prn pruritus. If pruritus not relieved after 2 hrs, consider nalbuphine 0.025 mg/kg/hr continuous drip (max 2 mg/hr).
		Signature ________ Printed Name ________ Date / Time ________

DO NOT WRITE IN BARCODE AREA CN 6-7400-950 EF (08/20/07) Page 2 of 5

CN 6-7400-950

TAB: ORDERS

Appendix IV. (Continued)

Children's
HOSPITAL • ST. LOUIS

ADMISSION ORDERS
VASO-OCCLUSIVE EPISODE
INTERMITTENT DOSE OPIOID
Recommended Age <7 years

ALL ORDERS MUST HAVE DATE, TIME WRITTEN, WRITER'S AND TRANSCRIBER'S LEGIBLE SIGNATURE (FIRST INITIAL, LAST NAME, TITLE) AND TRANSCRIPTION TIME. DIAGNOSIS AND ALLERGIES TO BE INCLUDED IN ALL ADMIT ORDERS.

Attending: **Unit:**

Diagnosis:

Allergies: (List or note NKA) **Height:** **Weight:**

Authorization is hereby given to dispense the generic or chemical equivalent unless otherwise indicated by the words "No Substitute."

Date	Time Written	Orders – Signatures – Transcription Times
		☐ Yes ☐ No **Asthma Orders:** *(If yes, complete below.)* 1. HR and RR pre- and post-albuterol treatments. 2. Measure peak flow pre- and post-albuterol treatments. 3. All nebulized medications and albuterol MDI to be given by Respiratory Therapist (RT). All other medications to be given by RN. 4. **Albuterol** ________ ml of nebulizer solution (5mg/ml) every _______ (2-4) hrs. 5. RT to wean albuterol treatments using Asthma Protocol. Call MD at time of each change. ☐ Yes ☐ No 6. Ipratropium (Atrovent®) 0.5 mg per 2.5 ml premixed nebulizer solution every 6 hrs. 7. *Systemic steroids* (ORDER ONE FORM): a. Methylprednisolone ______ mg IV every ______ hours, start __________ b. Prednisone TAB ______ mg po every ______ hours, start _________ c. Prednisolone LIQ ______ mg po every ______ hours, start _________ 8. Home asthma medications as follow: a. ____________________ b. ____________________ c. ____________________
		Bowel Regimen: Senna ☐ 1 mo-2 yrs 1.25 ml syrup po every hs (2.2 mg sennosides). Max dose 8.8 mg/day. ☐ 2 - < 6 yrs 2.5 ml syrup po every hs (4.4 mg sennosides). Max dose 8.8 mg/day. ☐ 6 - 12 yrs 1 tablet po every hs (8.8 mg sennosides). Max dose 17.2 mg/day. ☐ > 12 yrs 2 tablets po every hs (17.6 mg sennosides). Max dose 34.4 mg/day. *Patients receiving schedule opioids should be placed on a stimulant. If patient does not like Senna, can substitute Bisacodyl. **If no stool in 72 hrs, then double Senna dose and consider adding second agent.
		Other Medications: 1. ____________________ 2. ____________________ 3. ____________________ 4. ____________________
		Signature ________ Printed Name ________ Date / Time ________

DO NOT WRITE IN BARCODE AREA

CN 6-7400-950 EF (06/20/07) Page 3 of 5

CN 6-7400-950

TAB: ORDERS

Children's
HOSPITAL • ST. LOUIS
BJC HealthCare

ADMISSION ORDERS
VASO-OCCLUSIVE EPISODE
INTERMITTENT DOSE OPIOID
Recommended Age <7 years

ALL ORDERS MUST HAVE DATE, TIME WRITTEN, WRITER'S AND TRANSCRIBER'S LEGIBLE SIGNATURE (FIRST INITIAL, LAST NAME, TITLE) AND TRANSCRIPTION TIME. DIAGNOSIS AND ALLERGIES TO BE INCLUDED IN ALL ADMIT ORDERS.	
Attending:	**Unit:**
Diagnosis:	
Allergies: (List or note NKA)	**Height:** **Weight:**
Authorization is hereby given to dispense the generic or chemical equivalent unless otherwise indicated by the words "No Substitute."	

Date	Time Written	Orders – Signatures – Transcription Times
		Home Medications: ☐ Yes ☐ No Penicillin ☐ 2mo-3yr 125 mg po BID ☐ >3yr 250 mg po BID ☐ Yes ☐ No Folic Acid 1mg po every day 1. ____ 2. ____ 3. ____ 4. ____
		Adjuvant Therapies: ☐ Yes ☐ No 1. Referral to whirlpool therapy in PAWS. ☐ Yes ☐ No 2. Heating pad to bedside. 3. Contact Child Life regarding alternative coping strategies.
		Adjusting Pain Medications: 1. No wean in first 24 hrs except for adverse events such as respiratory depression, hallucinations or excessive sedation (non-responsiveness). 2. MD to assess breakthrough doses every 12 hrs and adjust maintenance dose appropriately.
		Other Guidelines: 1. Lights and Television off at 2100 on Sunday-Thursday for children less than 12 yrs. 2. Lights and Television off at 2300 on Sunday-Thursday for children older than 12 yrs. 3. Limit playroom time to no more than 45 minutes per day. 4. If patient hospitalized ≥ 3 days, then school age children should attend schoolroom Monday-Friday.
		Weaning Guidelines (MD to order): 1. Schedule wean in AM if patient slept through the night and is able to ambulate without severe pain. 2. Wean by 20% of original dose, preferably in the early AM (0600). 3. Continue to wean by 20% of original dose until dose is at 60% of original dose. 4. Re-evaluate before noon. If patient is comfortable, do not attempt second wean until 24 hrs later. Avoid weaning opioids in the afternoon or evening as pain is worse at night.
		Signature ____ Printed Name ____ Date / Time ____

DO NOT WRITE IN BARCODE AREA

CN 6-7400-950 EF (06/20/07) Page 4 of 5

CN 6-7400-950

TAB: ORDERS

Appendix IV. (Continued)

Children's
HOSPITAL • ST. LOUIS
BJC HealthCare

ADMISSION ORDERS
VASO-OCCLUSIVE EPISODE
INTERMITTENT DOSE OPIOID
Recommended Age <7 years

ALL ORDERS MUST HAVE DATE, TIME WRITTEN, WRITER'S AND TRANSCRIBER'S LEGIBLE SIGNATURE (FIRST INITIAL, LAST NAME, TITLE) AND TRANSCRIPTION TIME. DIAGNOSIS AND ALLERGIES TO BE INCLUDED IN ALL ADMIT ORDERS.

Attending: **Unit:**

Diagnosis:

Allergies: (List or note NKA) **Height:** **Weight:**

Authorization is hereby given to dispense the generic or chemical equivalent unless otherwise indicated by the words "No Substitute."

Date	Time Written	Orders – Signatures – Transcription Times
		Oral Conversion Guidelines (MD to order): 1. Cumulative dose of IV morphine received in previous 24 hrs x 3 = equivalent dose of oral morphine. Contact pharmacist for fentanyl and hydromorphone conversion. 2. Controlled Release Preparations: a. Oxycontin dose is equal to ½ of oral morphine divided po every 12 hrs. b. Morphine Sulfate Controlled Release (MS Contin) dose is ½ of oral morphine dose given po every 12 hrs. 3. Breakthrough Pain Medication: Morphine Sulfate immediate release (MSIR) or oxycodone to be given po every 3 to 4 hrs. The dose should be ¼ to ⅓ of oral dose of MS Contin or Oxycontin.
		Discharge Criteria: 1. Pain controlled on oral analgesics as assessed by patient/caregiver and physician. 2. Tolerating fluids by mouth and able to take po medications. 3. Afebrile for ≥ 24 hrs with negative blood cultures for ≥ 24 hrs if applicable. 4. Resolution of pulmonary symptoms and documentation of return to baseline saturations. 5. Stable hemoglobin (no drop ≥ 1.5 gm/dl in previous 24 hrs).
		Discharge Medication Guidelines: 1. Appropriate dose of long acting analgesic (Oxycontin or MSContin) if patient can take pills (cannot be crushed) and appropriate dose of short acting analgesic (Oxycodone MSIR, or Tylenol w/ codeine for children <5 yrs) for home use. Usually 30 doses of each. 2. Schedule long acting analgesic for 2 to 3 days at home. 3. Prescriptions for pain medications should be filled prior to discharge on **Hospital Day 2** including anticipated weekend or holiday discharges. Discharge medication doses should be calculated based on 60% of the 24 hour admission morphine requirement as per weaning guidelines. In case of weekend or holiday discharge, prescriptions must be picked up by the patient's caregiver prior to discharge during outpatient pharmacy hours.
		Other Discharge Guidelines: 1. Follow-up in 3 months for uncomplicated visit or 2 weeks if there are concerns. 2. Patient to resume school within 3 days of discharge.
		Signature / Printed Name / Date / Time

DO NOT WRITE IN BARCODE AREA

CN 6-7400-950 EF (08/20/07) Page 5 of 5

CN 6-7400-950

TAB: ORDERS

Appendix V

Staple

Children's

HOSPITAL • ST. LOUIS

BJC HealthCare

ADMISSION ORDERS
VASO-OCCLUSIVE EPISODE
FOR OPIOID PCA & INFUSIONS

ALL ORDERS MUST HAVE DATE, TIME WRITTEN, WRITER'S AND TRANSCRIBER'S LEGIBLE SIGNATURE (FIRST INITIAL, LAST NAME, TITLE) AND TRANSCRIPTION TIME. DIAGNOSIS AND ALLERGIES TO BE INCLUDED IN ALL ADMIT ORDERS.

Attending: **Unit:**

Diagnosis: Hgb S ___
Vaso-occlusive Episode
☐Y ☐N Asthma (Complete Asthma Section)
Other:

Allergies: (List or note NKA) **Height:** **Weight:**

Authorization is hereby given to dispense the generic or chemical equivalent unless otherwise indicated by the words "No Substitute."

Date	Time Written	Orders – Signatures – Transcription Times
		Condition:
		Nursing/Vitals: Temp, HR every _____ 2-4 hrs and RR every 2 hrs Continuous pulse oximetry. Notify HO for: HR > _______, RR > _______ or < _______, Temp ≥ 38.5°C, no UOP in > 8 hrs, worsening pain, sats ≤ 92% RA, or an increasing oxygen requirement.
		Respiratory: FiO_2 to keep sats ≥ 92%. Wean to room air for sats ≥ 92%. Incentive Spirometry: 10 breaths/hr while awake and recorded by nurse. ☐ Yes ☐ No Home nocturnal oxygen: ________________________ (if yes, amount).
		Diet:
		IV Fluids: D5½ NS with 20 meq KCL/L at ________ ml/hr. IVF + PO to equal 1500 to 2000 ml/m²/day. Reassess IVF needs every 24 hrs. May heplock IV and discontinue fluids if taking adequate po fluids.
		Activity: As tolerated. After 24 hours, begin ambulation for 10 minutes every 8 hrs.
		Laboratory: On Admission: CBC w/ diff, reticulocyte count if not done in ED or clinic. CBC w/ diff and reticulocyte count every day. BUN and creatinine on hospital day 1 for patients age 12 or older. ☐ Yes ☐ No Type and screen if hemoglobin ≥ 1 gm/dl below baseline. ☐ Yes ☐ No ALT, AST, fractionated bilirubin if concern for increased icterus.
		Signature Printed Name Date / Time

DO NOT WRITE IN BARCODE AREA

CN 6-7400-949 EF (06/29/07) Page 1 of 4

CN 6-7400-949

TAB: ORDERS

Appendix V. (Continued)

Children's
HOSPITAL • ST. LOUIS
BJC HealthCare

ADMISSION ORDERS
VASO-OCCLUSIVE EPISODE
FOR OPIOID PCA & INFUSIONS

ALL ORDERS MUST HAVE DATE, TIME WRITTEN, WRITER'S AND TRANSCRIBER'S LEGIBLE SIGNATURE (FIRST INITIAL, LAST NAME, TITLE) AND TRANSCRIPTION TIME. DIAGNOSIS AND ALLERGIES TO BE INCLUDED IN ALL ADMIT ORDERS.

Attending: **Unit:**

Diagnosis:

Allergies: (List or note NKA) **Height:** **Weight:**

Authorization is hereby given to dispense the generic or chemical equivalent unless otherwise indicated by the words "No Substitute."

Date	Time Written	Orders – Signatures – Transcription Times
		Pain Medications: Analgesics should be scheduled for all acute pain episodes. 1. Choose One: ☐ Morphine Sulfate ☐ Fentanyl ☐ Hydromorphone Select and complete standard PCA & Infusion orders including bowel regimen. ☐ Yes ☐ No 2. Ibuprofen 10 mg/kg __________mg po every 6 hrs unless contraindicated. ** If patient is unable to tolerate ibuprofen, consider acetaminophen at 15 mg/kg po every 6 hrs scheduled. Toradol po or IV not recommended.* 3. Patients on scheduled opioids should receive a bowel regimen. Order Senna on the standard PCA & Infusion Orders. *No stool in 72 hrs, double dose of Senna and consider adding a second agent.*
		☐ Yes ☐ No **Asthma Orders:** *(If yes, complete below.)* 1. HR and RR pre- and post-albuterol treatments. 2. Measure peak flow pre- and post-albuterol treatments. 3. All nebulized medications and albuterol MDI to be given by Respiratory Therapist (RT). All other medications to be given by RN. 4. Albuterol ________ ml of nebulizer solution (5mg/ml) every _______ (2-4) hrs. 5. RT to wean albuterol treatments using Asthma Protocol. Call MD at time of each change. ☐ Yes ☐ No 6. Ipratropium (Atrovent®) 0.5 mg per 2.5 ml premixed nebulizer solution every 6 hrs. 7. *Systemic steroids* (ORDER ONE FORM): a. Methylprednisolone ______ mg IV every ______ hours, start __________ b. Prednisone TAB ______ mg PO every ______ hours, start _________ c. Prednisolone LIQ ______ mg PO every ______ hours, start _________ 8. Home asthma medications as follow: a. ____________ b. ____________ c. ____________
		Other Medications: 1. ____________ 2. ____________ 3. ____________ 4. ____________
		____________ Signature ____________ Printed Name ____________ Date / Time

DO NOT WRITE IN BARCODE AREA CN 6-7400-949 EF (06/26/07) Page 2 of 4

CN 6-7400-949

TAB: ORDERS

Children's
HOSPITAL • ST. LOUIS
BJC HealthCare

ADMISSION ORDERS
VASO-OCCLUSIVE EPISODE
FOR OPIOID PCA & INFUSIONS

ALL ORDERS MUST HAVE DATE, TIME WRITTEN, WRITER'S AND TRANSCRIBER'S LEGIBLE SIGNATURE (FIRST INITIAL, LAST NAME, TITLE) AND TRANSCRIPTION TIME. DIAGNOSIS AND ALLERGIES TO BE INCLUDED IN ALL ADMIT ORDERS.

Attending: **Unit:**

Diagnosis:

Allergies: (List or note NKA) **Height:** **Weight:**

Authorization is hereby given to dispense the generic or chemical equivalent unless otherwise indicated by the words "No Substitute."

Date	Time Written	Orders – Signatures – Transcription Times
		Home Medications: ☐ Yes ☐ No 1. Penicillin: ☐ 2mos–3 yr 125 mg po BID ☐ >3 yr 250 mg po BID. ☐ Yes ☐ No 2. Folic Acid 1mg po every day. 3. ____ 4. ____
		Adjuvant Therapies: ☐ Yes ☐ No 1. Referral to whirlpool therapy in PAWS. ☐ Yes ☐ No 2. Heating pad to bedside. 3. Contact Child Life regarding alternative coping strategies.
		Adjusting Pain Medications: 1. No wean in first 24 hrs except for adverse events such as respiratory depression, hallucinations or excessive sedation (non-responsiveness). 2. MD to assess breakthrough doses every 12 hrs and adjust maintenance dose appropriately.
		Other Guidelines: 1. Lights and Television off at 2100 on Sunday-Thursday for children less than 12yrs. 2. Lights and Television off at 2300 on Sunday-Thursday for children 12 years and older. 3. Limit playroom time to no more than 45 minutes per day. 4. If patient hospitalized ≥ 3 days, then school age children should attend schoolroom Monday-Friday.
		Weaning Guidelines (MD to order): 1. Schedule wean in AM if patient slept through the night and is able to ambulate without severe pain. 2. Wean by 20% of original dose, preferably in the early AM (0600). 3. Continue to wean by 20% of original dose until dose is at 60% of original dose. 4. Re-evaluate before noon. If patient is comfortable, do not attempt second wean until 24 hrs later. Avoid weaning opioids in the afternoon or evening as pain is worse at night.
		Signature ____ Printed Name ____ Date / Time ____

DO NOT WRITE IN BARCODE AREA

CN 6-7400-949 EF (06/26/07) Page 3 of 4

CN 6-7400-949

TAB: ORDERS

Appendix I. (Continued)

Children's
HOSPITAL • ST. LOUIS
BJC HealthCare

ADMISSION ORDERS
VASO-OCCLUSIVE EPISODE
FOR OPIOID PCA & INFUSIONS

ALL ORDERS MUST HAVE DATE, TIME WRITTEN, WRITER'S AND TRANSCRIBER'S LEGIBLE SIGNATURE (FIRST INITIAL, LAST NAME, TITLE) AND TRANSCRIPTION TIME. DIAGNOSIS AND ALLERGIES TO BE INCLUDED IN ALL ADMIT ORDERS.

Attending: **Unit:**

Diagnosis:

Allergies: (List or note NKA) **Height:** **Weight:**

Authorization is hereby given to dispense the generic or chemical equivalent unless otherwise indicated by the words "No Substitute."

Date	Time Written	Orders – Signatures – Transcription Times

Oral Conversion Guidelines (MD to order):

1. Cumulative dose of IV morphine received in previous 24 hrs x 3 = equivalent dose of oral morphine. Contact pharmacist for fentanyl and hydromorphone conversion.
2. Controlled Release Preparations:
   a. Oxycontin dose is equal to ½ of oral morphine divided po every 12 hrs.
   b. Morphine Sulfate Controlled Release (MS Contin) dose is ½ of oral morphine dose given po every 12 hrs.
3. Breakthrough Pain Medication: Morphine Sulfate immediate release (MSIR) or oxycodone to be given po every 3 to 4 hrs. The dose should be ¼ to ⅓ of oral dose of MS Contin or Oxycontin.

Discharge Criteria:

1. Pain controlled on oral analgesics as assessed by patient/caregiver and physician.
2. Tolerating fluids by mouth and able to take po medications.
3. Afebrile for ≥ 24 hrs with negative blood cultures for ≥ 24 hrs if applicable.
4. Resolution of pulmonary symptoms and documentation of return to baseline saturations.
5. Stable hemoglobin (no drop ≥ 1.5 gm/dl in previous 24 hrs).

Discharge Medication Guidelines:

1. Appropriate dose of long acting analgesic (Oxycontin or MSContin) if patient can take pills (cannot be crushed) and appropriate dose of short acting analgesic (Oxycodone MSIR, or Tylenol w/ codeine for children <5 yrs) for home use. Usually 30 doses of each.
2. Schedule long acting analgesic for 2 to 3 days at home.
3. Prescriptions for pain medications should be filled prior to discharge on **Hospital Day 2** including anticipated weekend or holiday discharges. Discharge medication doses should be calculated based on 60% of the 24 hour admission morphine requirement as per weaning guidelines. In case of weekend or holiday discharge, prescriptions must be picked up by the patient's caregiver prior to discharge during outpatient pharmacy hours.

Other Discharge Guidelines:

1. Follow-up in 3 months for uncomplicated visit or 2 weeks if there are concerns.
2. Patient to resume school within 3 days of discharge.

Signature ______ Printed Name ______ Date / Time ______

DO NOT WRITE IN BARCODE AREA

CN 6-7400-949 EF (06/26/07) Page 4 of 4

CN 6-7400-949

TAB: ORDERS

References

[1] Frei-Jones MJ BA, Rogers ZR, Buchanan GR. Vaso-occlusive episodes in older children with sickle cell disease: emergency department management and pain assessment. J Peds 2007, in press.

[2] Panepinto JA, Brousseau DC, Hillery CA, Scott JP. Variation in hospitalizations and hospital length of stay in children with vaso-occlusive crises in sickle cell disease. Pediatr Blood Cancer 2005;44(2):182-6.

[3] Sloan PA, Montgomery C, Musick D. Medical student knowledge of morphine for the management of cancer pain. J Pain Symptom Manage 1998;15(6):359-64.

[4] Labbe E, Herbert D, Haynes J. Physicians' attitude and practices in sickle cell disease pain management. J Palliat Care 2005;21(4):246-51.

[5] Morrison RA. Update on sickle cell disease: incidence of addiction and choice of opioid in pain management. Pediatr Nurs 1991;17(5):503.

[6] Waldrop RD, Mandry C. Health professional perceptions of opioid dependence among patients with pain. Am J Emerg Med 1995;13(5):529-31.

[7] Tan WC, Ait-Khaled N. Dissemination and implementation of guidelines for the treatment of asthma. Int J Tuberc Lung Dis 2006;10(7):710-6.

[8] Grimshaw J, Eccles M, Tetroe J. Implementing clinical guidelines: current evidence and future implications. J Contin Educ Health Prof 2004;24 Suppl 1:S31-7.

[9] The Management of Sickle Cell Disease: National Institutes of Health, National Heart, Lung and Blood Institute, Division of Blood Diseases and Resources, 2002.

[10] National Newborn Screening Status Report. Austin: National Newborn Screening and Genetics Resource Center, 2007.

[11] Sickle cell research for treatment and cure. National Institutes of Health 2002; Publication No. 02-5214.

[12] Quinn CT, Miller ST. Risk factors and prediction of outcomes in children and adolescents who have sickle cell anemia. Hematol Oncol Clin North Am 2004;18(6):1339-54.

[13] Dampier C, Setty BNY, Eggleston B, Brodecki D, O'Neal P, Stuart M. Vaso-occlusion in children with sickle cell disease: clinical characteristics and biologic correlates. J Pediatr Hematol Oncol 2004;26(1077-4114):785-90.

[14] Platt OS, Thorington BD, Brambilla DJ, Milner PF, Rosse WF, Vichinsky E et al. Pain in sickle cell disease. N Engl J Med 1991;325(1):11-5.

[15] Ballas S. Sickle Cell Pain. Seattle: IASP Press, 1998.

[16] Battling Pain in Sickle Cell Disease: Fighting Racism, Stigma and Ignorance. In: Sohail Rana M, ed. Howard University, 2007.

[17] Nazaire H. www.defiers.com. In; 1997.

[18] Jacob E MC, Savedra M, Beyer JE, Treadwell M, Styles L. Changes in sleep, food intake and activity levels during acute painful episodes in children with sickle cell disease. J Pediatr Nurse 2006;21(1):23-34.

[19] Panepinto J, Brousseau D, Hillery C, Scott J. Variation in hospitalizations and hospital length of stay in children with vaso-occlusive crises in Sickle Cell Disease. Pediatr Blood Cancer 2005;44:182-6.

[20] Shapiro BS, Dinges DF, Carota Orne E, Bauer N, Reilly LB, Whitehouse WG et al. Home management of sickle cell-related pain in children and adolescents: a natural history and impact on school attendance. Pain 1995;61:139-44.

[21] King A, Herron S, McKinstry R, Bacak S, Armstrong M, White D et al. A multidisciplinary health care team's efforts to improve educational attainment in children with sickle-cell anemia and cerebral infarcts. J Sch Health 2006;76(1):33-7.

[22] Resar LM, Oski FA. Cold water exposure and vaso-occlusive crises in sickle cell anemia. J Pediatr 1991;118(3):407-9.

[23] Baum KF, Dunn DT, Maude GH, Serjeant GR. The painful crisis of homozygous sickle cell disease. A study of the risk factors. Arch Intern Med 1987;147(7):1231-4.

[24] Serjeant GR, Ceulaer CD, Lethbridge R, Morris J, Singhal A, Thomas PW. The painful crisis of homozygous sickle cell disease: clinical features. Br J Haematol 1994;87(3):586-91.

[25] Wright CS, Gardner E, Jr. A study of the role of acute infections in precipitating crises in chronic hemolytic states. Ann Intern Med 1960;52:530-7.

[26] Mohan J, Marshall JM, Reid HL, Thomas PW, Hambleton I, Serjeant GR. Peripheral vascular response to mild indirect cooling in patients with homozygous sickle cell (SS) disease and the frequency of painful crisis. Clin Sci (Lond) 1998;94(2):111-20.

[27] Smith WR, Coyne P, Smith VS, Mercier B. Temperature changes, temperature extremes, and their relationship to emergency department visits and hospitalizations for sickle cell crisis. Pain Manag Nurs 2003;4(3):106-11.

[28] Boyd JH, Moinuddin A, Strunk RC, DeBaun MR. Asthma and acute chest in sickle-cell disease. Pediatr Pulmonol 2004;38(3):229-32.

[29] Glassberg J, Spivey JF, Strunk R, Boslaugh S, DeBaun MR. Painful episodes in children with sickle cell disease and asthma are temporally associated with respiratory symptoms. J Pediatr Hematol Oncol 2006;28(8):481-5.

[30] Beyer JN, Simmons LE, Woods GM, Woods PM. A Chronology of pain and comfort in children with sickle cell disease. Arch Pediatr Adolesc Med 1999;153(9):913-20.

[31] Lieu TA, Quesenberry CP, Jr., Capra AM, Sorel ME, Martin KE, Mendoza GR. Outpatient management practices associated with reduced risk of pediatric asthma hospitalization and emergency department visits. Pediatrics 1997;100(3 Pt 1):334-41.

[32] Luffy R, Grove SK. Examining the validity, reliability, and preference of three pediatric pain measurement tools in African-American children. Pediatr Nurs 2003;29(1):54-9.

[33] Kokki H, Rasanen I, Reinikainen M, Suhonen P, Vanamo K, Ojanpera I. Pharmacokinetics of oxycodone after intravenous, buccal, intramuscular and gastric administration in children. Clin Pharmacokinet 2004;43(9):613-22.

[34] APS. Guideline for the Management of Acute and Chronic Pain in Sickle Cell Disease. Glenview, IL: American Pain Society; 1999.

[35] Silbergleit R, Jancis MO, McNamara RM. Management of sickle cell pain crisis in the emergency department at teaching hospitals. J Emerg Med 1999;17(4):625-30.

[36] Shapiro B, Cohen D, Howe C. Patient-controlled analgesia for sickle-cell-related pain. J Pain Symptom Manage 1993;8(1):22-8.

[37] Schechter N, Berrien F, Katz S. The use of patient-controlled analgesia in adolescents with sickle cell pain crisis: a preliminary report. J Pain Symptom Manage 1988;3(2):109-13.

[38] Robieux I, Kellner J, Coppes M, Shaw D, Brown E, Good C, et al. Analgesia in children with sickle cell crisis:comparison of intermittent opioids vs. continuous intravenous infusion of morphine and placebo controlled study of oxygen inhalation. Pediatr Hematol Oncol 1992;9:317-26.

[39] McDonald AJ, Cooper MG. Patient-controlled analgesia: an appropriate method of pain control in children. Paediatr Drugs 2001;3(4):273-84.

[40] Debaun MR, Derdeyn CP, McKinstry RC, 3rd. Etiology of strokes in children with sickle cell anemia. Ment Retard Dev Disabil Res Rev 2006;12(3):192-9.

[41] Brookoff D, Polomano R. Treating sickle cell pain like cancer pain. Ann Intern Med 1992;116(5):364-8.

[42] Dampier CD, Setty BN, Logan J, Ioli JG, Dean R. Intravenous morphine pharmacokinetics in pediatric patients with sickle cell disease. J Pediatr 1995;126(3):461-7.

[43] Christensen ML, Wang WC, Harris S, Eades SK, Wilimas JA. Transdermal fentanyl administration in children and adolescents with sickle cell pain crisis. J Pediatr Hematol Oncol 1996;18(4):372-6.

[44] Givens M, Rutherford C, Joshi G, Delaney K. Impact of an emergency department pain management protocol on the pattern of visits by patients with sickle cell disease. J Emerg Med 2007;32(3):239-43.

[45] Woods GM, Parson PM, Strickland DK. Efficacy of nalbuphine as a parenteral analgesic for the treatment of painful episodes in children with sickle cell disease. J Assoc Acad Minor Phys 1990;1(3):90-2.

[46] Buchanan I, Woodward M, Reed G. Opioid selection during sickle cell pain crisis and its impact on development of acute chest syndrome. Pediatr Blood Cancer 2005;45:716-24.

[47] Methadone and Cogeners, Goodman and Gilman's The Pharmacological Basis of Therapeutics. 9th ed, 1996.

[48] Gaedigk A, Bradford LD, Marcucci KA, Leeder JS. Unique CYP2D6 activity distribution and genotype-phenotype discordance in black Americans. Clin Pharmacol Ther 2002;72(1):76-89.

[49] Brousseau DC, McCarver DG, Drendel AL, Divakaran K, Panepinto JA. The effect of CYP2D6 polymorphisms on the response to pain treatment for pediatric sickle cell pain crisis. J Pediatr 2007;150(6):623-6.

[50] Meperidine and Cogeners, Goodman and Gilman's The Pharmacological Basis of Therapeutics. 9 th Ed, 1996.

[51] Marinella MA. Meperidine-induced generalized seizures with normal renal function. South Med J 1997;90(5):556-8.

[52] Nadvi SZ, Sarnaik S, Ravindranath Y. Low frequency of meperidine-associated seizures in sickle cell disease. Clin Pediatr (Phila) 1999;38(8):459-62.

[53] Hardwick WE GTMK, King WD, Lawley D. Effect of ketorolac in pediatric sickle cell vaso-occlusive pain crisis. Pedia Emerg Care 1999;15(3):179-82.

[54] Beiter JL SH, Chambliss R, Adamkiewicz T, Sullivan K. Intravenous ketorolac in the emergency department management of sickle cell pain and predictors of its effectiveness. Arch Pediatr Adolesc Med. 2001(155):496-500.

[55] Wright SW, Norris RL, Mitchell TR. Ketorolac for sickle cell vaso-occlusive crisis pain in the emergency department: lack of a narcotic-sparing effect. Ann Emerg Med 1992;21(8):925-8.

[56] Perlin E, Finke H, Castro O, Rana S, Pittman J, Burt R, et al. Enhancement of pain control with ketorolac tromethamine in patients with sickle cell vaso-occlusive crisis. Am J Hematol 1994;46(1):43-7.

[57] Simckes AM, Chen SS, Osorio AV, Garola RE, Woods GM. Ketorolac-induced irreversible renal failure in sickle cell disease: a case report. Pediatr Nephrol 1999;13(1):63-7.

[58] DeBaun MR. Fatal gastric hemorrhage in an adolescent patient with sickle cell anemia treated with ketoralac and ibuprofen. In; 2007.

[59] Jacobson S, Kopechy E, Joshi P, Babul N. Randomised trial of morphine for painful episodes of sickle cell disease in children. Lancet 1997;350:1359-61.

[60] Kopecky EA, Jacobson S, Joshi P, Koren G. Systemic exposure to morphine and the risk of acute chest syndrome in sickle cell disease. Clin Pharmacol Ther 2004;75(3):140-6.

[61] http://www.cancer.gov/. In: Institute NC, editor.; 2007.

[62] Ko MC, Song MS, Edwards T, Lee H, Naughton NN. The role of central mu opioid receptors in opioid-induced itch in primates. J Pharmacol Exp Ther 2004;310(1):169-76.

[63] Kjellberg F, Tramer MR. Pharmacological control of opioid-induced pruritus: a quantitative systematic review of randomized trials. Eur J Anaesthesiol 2001;18(6):346-57.

[64] de Stoutz ND, Bruera E, Suarez-Almazor M. Opioid rotation for toxicity reduction in terminal cancer patients. J Pain Symptom Manage 1995;10(5):378-84.

[65] Okomo U, Meremikwu MM. Fluid replacement therapy for acute episodes of pain in people with sickle cell disease. Cochrane Database Syst Rev 2007(2):CD005406.

[66] Frei-Jones MJ, Baxter AL, Rogers ZR, GR B. Vaso-Occlusive Episodes in Older Children with Sickle Cell Disease: Emergency Department Management and Pain Assessment. J Pediatr 2007;In press.

[67] Frush K, Ware RE, Kinney TR. Emergency department visits by children with sickle hemoglobinopathies: factors associated with hospital admission. Pediatr Emerg Care 1995;11(1):9-12.

[68] Haynes J, Jr., Allison RC. Pulmonary edema. Complication in the management of sickle cell pain crisis. Am J Med 1986;80(5):833-40.

[69] Bellet PS, Kalinyak KA, Shukla R, Gelfand MJ, Rucknagel DL. Incentive spirometry to prevent acute pulmonary complications in sickle cell diseases. N Engl J Med 1995;333(11):699-703.

[70] Strouse JJ, Takemoto CM, Keefer JR, Kato GJ, Casella JF. Corticosteroids and increased risk of readmission after acute chest syndrome in children with sickle cell disease. Pediatr Blood Cancer 2007.

[71] Strouse JJ, Hulbert ML, DeBaun MR, Jordan LC, Casella JF. Primary hemorrhagic stroke in children with sickle cell disease is associated with recent transfusion and use of corticosteroids. Pediatrics 2006;118(5):1916-24.

[72] Ballas SK, Lusardi M. Hospital readmission for adult acute sickle cell painful episodes: frequency, etiology, and prognostic significance. Am J Hematol 2005;79(1):17-25.

[73] Yang YM, Shah AK, Watson M, Mankad VN. Comparison of costs to the health sector of comprehensive and episodic health care for sickle cell disease patients. Public Health Rep 1995;110(1):80-6.

VII. Intellectual Disability

In: Children and Pain
Editors: P. Schofield and J. Merrick
ISBN 978-1-60876-020-6

Chapter 11

Children with intellectual disability and assessment of pain

Lynn M Breau**, PhD, RPsych
School of Nursing, Department of Pediatrics,
Department of Psychology, Dalhousie University and Complex Pain Team,
IWK Health Centre, Halifax, Nova Scotia, Canada

Abstract

Children with intellectual and developmental disabilities may be more susceptible to pain than typically developing children due to their medical conditions, treatment for those conditions that may cause pain, and greater risk for injury. Despite this, research to develop better pain management for them has lagged behind that for the general child population. In the past 15 years, research regarding pain assessment for this group has emerged.

This is important because pain assessment is the foundation of good pain management. Research at this time suggests that only a minority of children with an intellectual disability are capable of providing self-report using scales developed for typical children and that the abilities they do exhibit may be compromised during pain due to the nature of the experience. Because of this, observational measures of pain are recommended for most children in this population. Of those currently available, the Non-communicating Children's Pain Checklist appears to have the most sound psychometric properties for acute or chronic pain. It has also shown preliminary validity with adults, which can assist with ongoing assessment as children reach adulthood. Tools such as this only provide estimates of pain intensity, one dimension of pain. Thus, a comprehensive approach is recommended for ongoing pain, including assessment of pain intensity, location, temporal patterns. Changes in function and maladaptive behaviour should also be considered as they may reflect pain. A bio-ecological approach is encouraged, encompassing child, family and the social and cultural context of the child's pain.

* Correspondence: Lynn M Breau, Dalhousie University, 5869 University Avenue, Halifax, Nova Scotia, B3H 3J5, Canada. E-mail: lbreau@dal.ca

Introduction

Pain can be an adaptive part of everyday life. Its role is to warn us of injury or illness, so that action can be taken or help sought. Without pain, we risk repeated injuries and illness that can go unchecked. However, pain can also become maladaptive; as is the case when chronic pain persists long after tissue has healed. Pain's adaptive function is also curtailed when a person is unable to take action and has less ability to seek help, as is the case for infants and young children, the elderly with dementia, and those with intellectual or developmental disabilities.

In contrast to the main body of pain research, the bulk of research aimed at understanding the pain of children with intellectual or developmental disabilities has only emerged in the past decade, following about 10 years behind research of pain in typically developing children and infants. Because these children may have limited verbal abilities, they have been excluded from most studies of pain in which children are asked about their pain. Unlike research in the general population, however, pain research aimed at those with intellectual disabilities (ID) has emerged first for children, with studies of adult pain only recently being added. This may stem from the fact that methods used to assess pain in those with ID, and the issues involved in assessment, are more similar to those of typical children than typical adults.

Many children with ID suffer pain related to co-morbid physical disabilities and/or medical problems or to treatments for those problems (1). Poor detection of more common health problems may also lead to untreated pain (2), and injuries are also more common in this group (3), especially those who are mobile (4). Research also suggests that pain has substantial impacts on children's daily function (5) and may lead to unwanted behaviour such as self-injury (6). This mounting body of evidence, therefore, makes it clear that pain presents a serious problem for children with ID.

Families and caregivers of these children are also affected by a child's pain. Parents report that they struggle with healthcare professionals when seeking care for pain. They believe professionals have difficulty assessing and treating their child's pain and that their child's pain is treated differently than that of typical children (7). Some parents report a feeling of isolation and inordinate responsibility because professionals, who have difficulty with treating their child, refer decisions back to the parent (2). Parents also report anger that their child must suffer pain in addition to their other problems, but also a sense of helplessness and emotional turmoil (8). These accounts highlight the fact that the children's suffering due to pain also impacts their family.

Pain assessment as a foundation for pain management

Pain assessment is the foundation of good pain management, so it is the key to improving care for children with ID. In many cases, treatments for the pain these children experience do exist, but are not used because pain remains undetected. The effectiveness of treatments may also be questioned because pain is not monitored, sometimes leading to the abandonment of attempts to manage the child's pain. Good pain assessment is, therefore, crucial at all stages of pain management; from detection, to monitoring treatment, to prevention in situations where pain may occur, such as during medical procedures.

Self-report is considered the "gold standard" for pain assessment. For self-report to be appropriate, however, the individual with pain must be capable of appraising their pain and of communicating that internal experience to others. For many people with ID this isn't possible. In the absence of self-report, observational tools can be used to measure an individual's pain based on overt behaviour. This approximation is usually an underestimate, since not all aspects of the pain experience are expressed in overt behaviour. However, correspondence between observational estimates and self-report can be good under the correct circumstances.

Accounting for biased observers

One requirement for good assessment is that biases or preconceived beliefs of those observing pain behaviour not cloud objective evaluation of the evidence they may see or hear from someone with pain. This can be problematic for children with ID because some reports have suggested that people with ID are insensitive or indifferent to pain (9) and this belief could lead to underestimates of pain or discounting of potential pain. However, these suggestions have been based primarily on anecdotal reports or un-validated pain assessment methods. In contrast, research suggests that some adults believe that children with ID may over-react to pain (10), which could also lead to less than adequate management if parents feel the reaction does not reflect the true severity of the child's pain. The use of a sound assessment tool can reduce the likelihood that evaluation is tainted with preconceived beliefs, but cannot eliminate the potential for minimizing the importance of pain for children with ID, regardless of whether the observer believes these children over- or under-react to pain. For example, in a study by Fanurik et al., 29% of parents reported that they believe their child's pain is treated differently solely because of their ID (7). For the professional, awareness of their personal beliefs regarding pain in this group may be the best guard against unintentional influence on clinical care.

Evaluating psychometrics of assessment tools

A second requirement for good pain assessment is that the observational pain tool being used has proven psychometric properties. This may be more important with this population because of biases and that professionals may have relatively less experience with the way these children show pain. Pain intensity is the focus of most pain tools, and reflects only one component of the pain experience. Nonetheless, it is a useful parameter clinically and appears to be the most easily quantified quality of the multidimensional pain experience. An understanding of the key psychometric aspects of a pain tool is especially important when looking at those for use with children with ID. Many of the tools that exist are still under study, meaning that ongoing research can show limitations or extensions of their use. Thus, professionals should keep basic psychometric concepts in mind when deciding which tool to use.

A sound pain assessment tool must be both valid and reliable. A valid tool specifically measures the desired construct and nothing else. In the case of pain, that means ensuring that the tool measures pain specifically, not anxiety or distress or illness. Validity is tested by comparing the scores from a tool to other measures of pain taken at the same time, either by other observers or from the individual who has pain in the form of self-report. It can also be determined by comparing scores during pain to those when pain is absent or after pain has been treated. A reliable tool provides the same score each time it is used or when used by different people. Pain assessment tools should provide consistently low scores when people do not have pain and consistently higher scores when they do have pain. If the tool is designed for use by multiple observers, then scores from these should not differ substantially. Validity and reliability are context-dependent; they may vary due to the setting (e.g. hospital or home), the person completing the tool (caregiver or family member), the type of pain and context of pain (e.g. chronic pain versus acute procedural pain) and the person who has pain (adult versus child, intellectual disability alone versus intellectual and physical disabilities). This means research must be conducted to evaluate the validity and reliability of a tool in numerous contexts before it can be considered valid and reliable for general use. Until that time, it should only be considered sound in those circumstances in which it was tested or in very similar ones.

Pain assessment methods

Early research regarding pain in people with ID

Although the bulk of recent research regarding pain in children with ID has focused on assessment, early research in this area focussed primarily on individual cases or on the apparent differences in response to pain by people with ID (11,12).

The first study to show pain leads to consistent behaviours appeared in 1965 (13). Reynell provided evidence that children with ID experience pain under circumstances most children would be expected to have pain, following surgery, that their pain behaviour was observable, and that it did not vary due to level of impairment. Cases studies predominated the literature for 30 years after Reynell's first report (14-16). Then, in 1995, Giusiano et al (17) recorded pain behaviour observed during a physical exam by 100 individuals aged 2 to 33 years in a long-term care facility. This seminal study provided the first indication that a set of common pain behaviours could be observed and aggregated into a basic assessment tool for people with ID. Since then, two main approaches have been undertaken in efforts to improve assessment for this group.

On the one hand, studies have explored whether tools designed for typical children are valid when used with children who have ID. On the other, studies have been conducted to develop new instruments, most often based on empirical evidence for observable pain responses by the children.

Pain assessment tools designed for typical children

Facial Expression. Studies with children with ID have reported differing results when trying to use facial expression to detect pain. In the first study published, Oberlander et al (18) found no significant change in facial reaction to pain during a mock and real immunization for eight adolescents with spastic quadriplegia (18). Similarly, Hadden et al (19) observed no change in facial expression during home physiotherapy exercises in 19 children with cerebral palsy, although pain ratings using the Non-communicating Children's Pain Checklist did increase during stretches. In contrast, Nader et al (20) did report increased facial activity in 21 children with autism when they were observed during intravenous needles, as well as greater facial activity relative to controls. These three studies used the Child Facial Coding System (21), which has shown some validity with typical children (22,23). However, the differences in results here raise questions as to whether this research tool has potential for children with ID. Mercer and Glenn (24) found facial response in 8 infants with developmental delay who were receiving immunizations did change with needle insertion. Facial expression was also not diminished, but was more diffuse than in a comparison group of 30 infants without ID, when they used the Maximally Discriminative Facial Movement Coding System. Thus, the tool used may underlie differences in results among these studies. However, there is clearly a great deal of work to be done in this area before clinical use of any facial expression tool is feasible. Not only must more support for their validity be found. But also, most current systems are time-consuming and coded from videotape, making bedside application impractical.

Multidimensional tools

Although the development of observational tools to assess pain in people with ID has proceeded quickly since the 1990s, some research of tools designed for typical children has also occurred in parallel. One group examined the validity of the FLACC scale (Faces, Legs, Acitvity, Cry, Consolability) for measuring pain in children with ID after surgery (25). Revisions improved the reliability (26), but cut-offs developed with the original scale may no longer be appropriate for the revised scale because mean scores differed after the changes. The revised scale also allows for personalization of items by a caregiver or parent. However, it is not clear how this would affect cut-off values. More research is needed before the FLACC is used clinically for people with ID.

Soetenga et al (27) used the University of Wisconsin Children's Hospital Pain Scale with 74 children admitted to hospital, 15 of whom were over age 3 years, but nonverbal. This scale contains four subscales: Vocal, Facial, Behavior and Body Movement. Scores were significantly lower after analgesic administration and inter-rater reliability was excellent. However, subgroup analyses for the nonverbal children in the sample are not provided, so it is difficult to conclude whether the psychometrics presented would be similar had the scores for the subgroup been examined separately.

Most recently, Solodiuk and Curley (28) suggested the use of an individualized visual analogue scale (VAS) for children with severe cognitive impairments. A caregiver is asked to provide descriptors for the 0 and 10 anchors and points between. They report this has worked well clinically, but have not yet reported data on the validity or reliability of this measure. Overall, there is not convincing evidence that the tools above are satisfactory for children with ID. Although further research may provide additional evidence to support their use clinically, they not be used clinically at this time.

Self-report pain tools

Since self-report is the "gold standard" of pain assessment, it is important to consider it as a possibility when assessing pain in individuals with ID. Fanurik et al (29) were the first to explore the self-report abilities of children with borderline to profound ID. They found only half of children with borderline ID and less than 30% of the group with mild ID could pass tests indicating they understood order and magnitude, two concepts encompassed in commonly used scales of pain intensity. Benini et al (30) found the number of children in their study who chose a rating indicating pain after venepuncture varied depending on whether a standard or modified scale was used. The scales they included were the Eland Color Scale (31) and an adaptation of that scale, and the Facial Affective Scale (32), along with a modified version. This is contrasted by several studies that have asked children or adults with ID to rate hypothetical pain situations using various types of pain scales (33-35). They have found higher rates of successful use of self-report pain rating scales that the studies conducted by Benini or Fanurik's groups. This discrepancy suggests that people with ID may appear more capable when rating hypothetical pain than they are in real-life pain situations. Research with the general population indicates cognitive abilities are usually reduced during pain, and those with ID are not likely exempt from this effect. In fact, Benini et al. reports fear reduced success in their study (30). This is relevant to clinical situations, where professionals often ask children to "practice" using a scale by rating hypothetical events, such as scraping a knee. The child's ability in using the tool for these trials may not reflect her ability during actual pain.

Observational tools designed for children with ID

Echelle Douleur Enfant San Salvador (DESS). Since their first study published in 1995, Collignon and Giusiano and their group (36) have continued their development of the DESS. In a second study, they reduced the original 22 behaviours to 10 items and report that a score of 2 indicates "pain is possible", while a score of 6 indicates "definite pain needing treatment" (36). A strength of this scale is that it was based on research with children and adults, making it useful across age groups. However, several weaknesses undermine the scale's psychometrics. Overlap among items means that crying behaviours carry an inordinate weight in scoring and some items incorporate the subjective opinion of caregivers. Unfortunately, the DESS is also designed so that items are rated in relation to the individual's typical behavior. This may be possible, or even preferred in some situations, but makes the tool less valid when observers do not know the person's typical behaviour. Using change from typical behavior also means that scores cannot be used across situations (e.g. home versus school/hospital) as children often exhibit pain differently in hospital where they feel more inhibited in front of staff. Finally, validation of the DESS was conducted in French. Caution should be taken in using those cut-off values if using an English version of the scale until systematic translation and validation in English is completed. Cultural and language differences can impact both pain behavior displayed and our perception of pain behavior.

The Paediatric Pain Profile (PPP)

This scale was developed through interviews with 21 caregivers of children with ID (37). From an original pool of 56 items, a set of 20 was selected. Inter-rater reliability between parents and a caregiver was reported to be good. Scores also decreased significantly after analgesics were given. Although a cut-off score is provided, it only identifies moderate pain. In a second study of a subgroup of the original sample, scores in a home setting were compared during videotaped daily activities thought to be painful for children with chronic pain conditions but not those without chronic pain (38). However, the cut-off varied slightly from the first study and a different method of computing scores was used. One positive attribute of the scale is that the developers have created a package that caregivers can complete to document their child's baseline behaviour when he is pain free and behaviour during common pains. This might be particularly helpful in cases where children have multiple conditions that cause chronic or recurrent pain, as it might help to untangle the temporal patterns of specific pains. However, with only two studies to date, some change in the cut-off values, data from only one population and no data in a hospital setting, the Paediatric Pain Profile needs more research support before it is used widely for on the spot pain assessment.

The Non-communicating Children's Pain Checklists (NCCPC's)

In the mid-1990's, a series of studies began that reported the development, testing and revision of the Non-communicating Children's Pain Checklist. The original scale included yes/no responses to 30 items in seven categories: Vocal, Eating/Sleeping, Social/Personality, Facial Expression, Activity, Body and Limbs, and Physiological (39). In the original study, which included children and adults, no differences in scores were found due to age (3 to 44 years) of the person with ID. A further study of the NCCPC–Postoperative Version (NCCPC-PV) investigated its use for postoperative pain (40). Items from the Eating/Sleeping subscale were excluded and more detailed responses from observers were added, such that they now provided ratings to indicate whether each item was observed "not at all", just a little", "fairly often" or "very often" during 10 minute pre- and postoperative observations of 24 children. A cut-off score for moderate to severe pain (equivalent to 3+ out of 10 on a 10 cm visual analogue scale) was set at 11 and detected 88% of cases. Later, a score of 6 to 10 was developed to detect mild pain (< 3 /10 on a 10 cm visual analogue scale of pain), with 75% accuracy. Caregivers' (parents and primary caregivers) and researcher' total scores increased after surgery, as would be expected. Total scores between the two observers were also significantly correlated, indicating good inter-rater reliability. This is especially important , because it indicates scores from an observer who is unfamiliar with the child (researcher) are valid.

The original NCCPC was also revised for the home setting, and renamed the NCCPC-Revised (NCCPC-R). The 30 items were retained, but the frequency scoring used for the NCCPC-PV was adopted. It was re-examined in a home setting with a larger sample than the first study (39), and based on two-hour observations of children. Scores for children who had pain during the observations were compared to scores for children who did not have pain. A total score of 7 detected pain in 84% of cases. The results also indicated total NCCPC-R scores were consistent across the two episodes of pain, as were the number of items children displayed. This is important because it has been suggested that children with ID show pain inconsistently. This result negates that; revealing that their pain response is consistent between two episodes of pain due to two different causes.

The NCCPC's were specifically designed for children who had very limited verbal abilities due to their ID. However, Hadden and von Baeyer have also used the NCCPC-R with children with cerebral palsy with varying levels of verbal abilities. Parents identified items from the checklist that occurred when their child had pain. The reported presence of 24 items from the NCCPC-R did not vary due to the children's communication ability (41). In a subsequent study by the same authors, 129 children with cerebral palsy who had a wide range of verbal abilities, were observed during home physiotherapy exercises that were expected to cause pain (19). Although children's facial expression did not change significantly during active stretching, scores on the NCCPC-PV were significantly higher. Thus, there is some evidence that the NCCPC's may be valid for higher functioning children with physical impairments. Breau et al. also examined whether the NCCPC-R is valid for children who display self-injurious behavior (6). This is a concern because, despite evidence to the contrary, some believe that these children may be insensitive to pain. There were no significant differences in NCCPC-R total scores for observed episodes of pain in children with (n = 44) and without (n = 57) a history of ongoing self-injury. The results also suggested that children who had chronic pain might show a different pattern of self-injury, suggesting self-injurious behavior might be a reaction to pain in some children.

The NCCPC's have also been translated into several languages. Although a recent study of 24 children in a rehabilitation hospital indicated good reliability and validity when used by parents or caregivers, it also suggested a cut-off score of 5 was more appropriate for the Swiss-German version (42). This highlights the need for validating translated scales, because interpretations of items may differ due to language constraints or cultural factors. Children may also display behaviour differently depending on cultural norms regarding appropriate pain expression. A French translation of the NCCPC- PV, developed in Canada and France, is currently being validated in hospitals in Canada and France. This study also incorporated a change in the observation time needed, in an attempt to improve feasibility of the NCCPC-PV in a clinical setting. Observations were reduced from the 10 minutes of previous research, to 5 minutes. Preliminary data for the «Grille d'Évaluation de la douleur - déficience intellectuelle» with 77 participants aged 3 to 57 suggest scores increase after surgery and may be similar to those found with the English version (43). Mean pre-operative scores were below 7.0, while mean post-operative scores were over 14.0. Further detailed analyses will reveal whether the scores differ due to age (child/adult) or culture.

Very recently, the NCCPC–R has also been used with 159 adults with ID who received vaccinations (44). Although scores differed prior to the immunization due to level of ID, they increased significantly after vaccination regardless of level of ID. New data, using the NCCPC-R for chronic pain in 17 adults with an average age of 42 years, reveals mean total NCCPC-R scores of 4.8 (SD = 5.2) when pain is absent and 32.3 (SD = 13.8) when pain is present (Burkitt and Breau, manuscript submitted for publication). This study also incorporated a reduced observation time of 5 minutes. Although further research is needed to provide more psychometric evidence for use of the NCCPC's with adults, these early studies suggest that the NCCPC's have the potential to be used throughout the lifespan, which can ease transition to adult care.

Summary

There are more similarities than differences among scales created for children and adults with ID. This supports the argument that pain behaviour is consistent in this population and that a standardized scale can be developed for children with ID. The basis on which to choose a scale then becomes a matter of the amount of research supporting the tool's psychometric properties. To date, the NCCPC's have the most evidence to support their use clinically for children with ID and there is some data to suggest that they may continue to be used as youth transition to adulthood, which may be helpful in documenting long-term or recurrent pain problems that can span years. The NCCPC's have been used across a number of studies by different research groups. These have included children and adults and have taken place in home, hospital and residential facilities, suggesting the NCCPC- R and NCCPC- PV can be used widely within the population of children and adults with ID. For current clinical use, the NCCPC-PV is recommended because its shorter observation period (currently 10 minutes) makes it more feasible. Cut-offs are available for mild pain (Total score = 6-10) and moderate to severe pain (Total score = 11+).

Putting research into practice

Parents have identified pain as an area of concern for their children who cannot communicate verbally (45). They also express concern that some professionals may discount their reports that their child has pain (2) and that their child's pain is treated differently than that of typical children (7). In interview studies, parents also report that familiarity with their child is required to assess their child's pain (2,8). No professional would argue the fact that each child is unique, whether or not she has ID. However, parents' beliefs about the inability of professionals to manage their child's pain may reflect assumptions based on past experience in which professionals failed in attempts to discern pain due to lack of training, little literature to provide guidance, and the unavailability of structured tools to help them to assess pain. The landscape has changed dramatically in the past 10 years, with increased research and awareness of issues regarding pain assessment for this particular group.

Among the important advancements that have been made is the understanding that variation in children's pain behavior does not preclude the use of validated measures that have been empirically and scientifically evaluated with this population. When provided with information in a structured way, or using a validated tool, observers who are unfamiliar with children with ID may provide very reliable judgments. For example, the good inter-rater reliability between parents and a researcher reported by Breau et al. (40) suggests use of a structured tool may facilitate agreement and reduce the impact of preconceived beliefs during pain assessment. Professionals may also be very adept at putting aside preconceived beliefs regarding a group, when dealing with one child in a clinical situation using a tool that helps them to structure their evaluation.

Thus, pain assessment for children with ID should follow the same principles as that for other groups. Self-report is always the preferred method of obtaining information about pain intensity. However, it is advisable to test the child's abilities to understand the underlying concepts when possible. Training a child in how to use a scale, by having him rate hypothetical situations (46) may improve his skills if he understands the concepts necessary for using a self-report scale. However, the possibility that the child's abilities may be reduced during actual pain should be kept in mind. The NCCPC-PV should be used when self-report is not possible, whether for chronic or acute pain. It has fewer items that the NCCPC-R and a shorter (10 minute versus 2 hour) observation time, and new data is suggesting that information regarding eating and sleeping patterns (included in the NCCPC-R) may not be necessary for accurate pain assessment. These aspects of behaviour are more difficult to assess because they cannot be judged over a short time frame, and they may be more difficult for observers who are unfamiliar with a child to evaluate, since they require some knowledge of the child's typical eating and sleeping patterns. When chronic or recurrent pain is suspected, multiple applications of the NCCPC-PV can provide information regarding the temporal pattern of pain and can help to disentangle behaviour changes due to pain from those due to factors such as illness or sleep problems. Records of a child's pain history, using a format such as that provided with the Paediatric Pain Profile (37) can also be useful for helping to untangle multiple sources of pain and for developing a dossier that can be used to help with diagnosis of pain problems.

Although ratings of pain intensity may be sufficient to inform management of acute pain due to procedures or injury, additional information may be helpful for cases of chronic pain. Any information regarding pain quality and location that can be collected will assist with diagnosis. Some research suggests that self-injury may also be a cue, not only of pain presence, but also of pain location and temporal pattern (6). Changes in a person's functioning may also help assess pain presence, as well as alert caregivers to potential skill losses that may occur due to pain and reduce daily functioning and independence (5).

Pain is multidimensional, affecting multiple areas of a person's life and having sensory, cognitive and emotional components. Bronfenbrenner's Bio-ecological Model (47) has been proposed as a model for comprehensive pain management for typical children with chronic pain (48). This model may serve children with ID just as well, since it is based on the premise that children are evolving beings, each with their own growth trajectory. Thus, it allows for the fact that children with ID may differ in their developmental path from typical peers. The model also incorporates the idea that each child's unique set of environments impact the pain experience, which is very important to consider for this particular group of children who may be exposed to situations and experiences not common for most children, such as residential care or repeated medical procedures or hospitalizations. The model also accounts for the fact that pain itself becomes part of the child's environment, interacting with the child, family and society and changing their dynamic relations. Finally, the model emphasizes the importance of the child's internal characteristics, among which is her ability to comprehend pain and its causes and treatments. Children with ID may have limited abilities to understand abstract aspects of pain or to follow the logic of treatments, which may affect their willingness to report pain or to cooperate with treatment. At the same time, they may have extensive experience with pain and many memories of painful experiences, which can add to emotional reactions to pain. This complex internal environment is not inconsequential and should be taken into account with each child. Discussion with a child regarding his experience should be frequent, so that his perceptions can be taken into account when making treatment decisions. Information should not be kept from him. This could lead to a lack of trust and an attempt by him to hide pain. Finally, all information and assessment methods should be appropriate to the child's cognitive or mental age and not based on standards for the general child population, chronological age, or assumptions that a long history of pain has increased the child's comprehension of pain. All pain assessment activities should be coordinated within a comprehensive pain management plan that should be from a multi-disciplinary approach whenever possible. Untreated pain can lead to mood and anxiety problems, maladaptive behaviour and functional impairments for people with ID, a group who can sorely afford any additional burdens to reaching their fullest potential. Research regarding pain in children has advanced a great deal in the past 15 years, but much is still unknown, particularly about the long-term consequences for these children who already have burdens that can hinder development. Pain is an unnecessary burden in most cases, because actions could be taken to prevent or treat it. Because of its pivotal role in pain management, good pain assessment is vital to any attempt to improve care for this vulnerable group of children.

Acknowledgments

The author is supported by a New Investigator Salary Award from the Canadian Institutes of Health Research.

References

[1] Breau LM, Camfield CS, McGrath PJ, Finley GA. The incidence of pain in children with severe cognitive impairments. Arch Pediatr Adolesc Med 2003;157(12):1219-26.

[2] Hunt A, Mastroyannopoulou K, Goldman A, Seers K. Not knowing--the problem of pain in children with severe neurological impairment. Int J Nurs Stud 2003; 40(2):171-83.

[3] Braden K, Swanson S, Di Scala C. Injuries to children who had preinjury cognitive impairment: a 10-year retrospective review. Arch Pediatr Adolesc Med 2003; 157(4):336-40.
[4] Breau LM, Camfield CS, McGrath PJ, Finley GA. Risk factors for pain in children with severe cognitive impairments. Dev Med Child Neurol 2004; 46(6):364-71.
[5] Breau LM, Camfield CS, McGrath PJ, Finley GA. Pain's impact on adaptive functioning. J Intellect Disabil Res 2007; 51(Pt 2):125-34.
[6] Breau LM, Camfield CS, Symons FJ, Bodfish JW, Mackay A, Finley GA et al. Relation between pain and self-injurious behavior in nonverbal children with severe cognitive impairments. J Pediatr 2003; 142(5):498-503.
[7] Fanurik D, Koh JL, Schmitz ML, Harrison RD, Conrad TM. Children with cognitive impairment: Parent report of pain and coping. J Dev Behav Pediatr 1999;20(4):228-34.
[8] Carter B, McArthur E, Cunliffe M. Dealing with uncertainty: parental assessment of pain in their children with profound special needs. J Adv Nurs 2002;38(5):449-57.
[9] Biersdorff KK. Pain insensitivity and indifference: alternative explanations for some medical catastrophes. Ment Retard 1991; 29(6):359-62.
[10] Breau LM, MacLaren J, McGrath PJ, Camfield CS, Finley GA. Caregivers' beliefs regarding pain in children with cognitive impairment: relation between pain sensation and reaction increases with severity of impairment. Clin J Pain 2003;19(6):335-44.
[11] Couston TA. Indifference to pain in low-grade mental defectives. Br Med J 1954;1(4871):1128-9.
[12] Stengel E, Oldham AJ, Ehrenberg AS. Reactions of low-grade mental defectives to pain. J Ment Sci 1958;104(435):434-8.
[13] Reynell JK. Post-operative disturbances observed in children with cerebral palsy. Dev Med Child Neurol 1965;7(4):360-76.
[14] Mette F, Abittan J. Essais d'évaluation de la douleur chez le polyhandicapé. Annales Kinésithérapie 1988;15:101-4.
[15] L'automutilation: expression de la douleur chez le sujet deficient mental profond. La Douleur de l'Enfant Quelles Resposes?; 92 A.D. Dec 15; Paris: UNESCO, 1992. [French]
[16] Collignon P, Giusiano B, Porsmoguer E, Jimeno ME, Combe JC. Difficultes du diagnostic de la douleur chez l'enfant polyhandicape. Ann Pediatr 1995;42(2):123-6. [French]
[17] Giusiano B, Jimeno MT, Collignon P, Chau Y. Utilization of a neural network in the elaboration of an evaluation scale for pain in cerebral palsy. Methods Inf Med 1995;34:498-502.
[18] Oberlander TF, Gilbert CA, Chambers CT, O'Donnell ME, Craig KD. Biobehavioral responses to acute pain in adolescents with a significant neurologic impairment. Clin J Pain 1999;15:201-9.
[19] Hadden KL, von Baeyer CL. Global and Specific Behavioral Measures of Pain in Children With Cerebral Palsy. Clin J Pain 2005; 21(2):140-6.
[20] Nader R, Oberlander TF, Chambers CT, Craig KD. Expression of pain in children with autism. Clin J Pain 2004;20(2):88-97.
[21] Chambers CT, Cassidy KL, McGrath PJ, Gilbert CA, Craig KD. Child facial coding system: A manual. Nova Scotia: Dalhousie Univ, Univ British Columbia, 1996.
[22] Breau LM, McGrath PJ, Craig KD, Santor D, Cassidy KL, Reid GJ. Facial expression of children receiving immunizations: A principal components analysis of the Child Facial Coding System. Clin J Pain 2001;17(2):178-86.
[23] Gilbert CA, Lilley CM, Craig KD, McGrath PJ, Court C, Bennett SM et al. Postoperative pain expression in preschool children: Validation of the child facial coding system. Clin J Pain 1999; 15(3):192-200.
[24] Mercer K, Glenn S. The expression of pain in infants with developmental delays. Child Care Health Dev 2004;30(4):353-60.
[25] Voepel-Lewis T, Merkel S, Tait AR, Trzcinka A, Malviya S. The reliability and validity of the Face, Legs, Activity, CRY, Consolability observational tool as a measure of pain in children with cognitive impairment. Anesth Analg 2002;95:1224-9.

[26] Malviya S, Voepel-Lewis T, Burke C, Merkel S, Tait AR. The revised FLACC observational pain tool: improved reliability and validity for pain assessment in children with cognitive impairment. Pediatr Anesth 2006;16(3):258-65.
[27] Soetenga D, Pellino TA, Frank J. Assessment of the validity and reliability of the University of Wisconsin Children's Hospital pain scale for preverbal and nonverbal children. Pediatr Nurs 1999; 25(6):670-6.
[28] Solodiuk J, Curley MA. Pain assessment in nonverbal children with severe cognitive impairments: the Individualized Numeric Rating Scale (INRS). J Pediatr Nurs 2003;18(4):295-9.
[29] Fanurik D, Koh JL, Harrison RD, Conrad TM, Tomerlin C. Pain assessment in children with cognitive impairment: An exploration of self-report skills. Clin Nurs Res 1998;7(2):103-24.
[30] Benini F, Trapanotto M, Gobber D, Agosto C, Carli G, Drigo P et al. Evaluating pain induced by venipuncture in pediatric patients with developmental delay. Clin J Pain 2004;20(3):156-63.
[31] Eland JM. The child who is hurting. Semin Oncol Nurs 1985; 1(2):116-22.
[32] McGrath PA, deVeber LL, Hearn MJ. Multidimensional pain assessment in children. In: Fields HR, Dubner R, Cevero F, eds. Advances in pain research and therapy, Vol 9. New York: Raven Press, 1985.
[33] Zabalia M, Jacquet D, Breau LM. Rôle du niveau verbal sur l'expression et l'évaluation de la douleur chez des sujets déficients intellectuals. Doul et Analg 2005;2:65-70. [French]
[34] Boldingh EJ, Jacobs-van der Bruggen MA, Lankhorst GJ, Bouter LM. Assessing pain in patients with severe cerebral palsy: development, reliability, and validity of a pain assessment instrument for cerebral palsy. Arch Phys Med Rehabil 2004; 85(5):758-66.
[35] Bromley J, Emerson E, Caine A. The development of a self-report measure to assess the location and intensity of pain in people with intellectual disabilities. J Intellect Disabil Res 1998;42:72-80.
[36] Collignon P, Giusiano B. Validation of a pain evaluation scale for patients with severe cerebral palsy. Eur J Pain 2001;5(4):433-42.
[37] Hunt A, Goldman A, Seers K, Crichton N, Mastroyannopoulou K, Moffat V et al. Clinical validation of the paediatric pain profile. Dev Med Child Neurol 2004;46(1):9-18.
[38] Hunt A, Wisbeach A, Seers K, Goldman A, Crichton N, Perry L et al. Development of the paediatric pain profile: role of video analysis and saliva cortisol in validating a tool to assess pain in children with severe neurological disability. J Pain Symptom Manage 2007; 33(3):276-89.
[39] Breau LM, McGrath PJ, Camfield C, Rosmus C, Finley GA. Preliminary validation of an observational pain checklist for persons with cognitive impairments and inability to communicate verbally. Dev Med Child Neurol 2000;42(9):609-16.
[40] Breau LM, Finley GA, McGrath PJ, Camfield CS. Validation of the Non-Communicating Children's Pain Checklist - Postoperative version. Anesthesiology 2002;96(3):528-35.
[41] Hadden KL, von Baeyer CL. Pain in children with cerebral palsy: common triggers and expressive behaviors Pain 2002;99(1-2):281-8.
[42] Kleinknecht M. [Reliability and validity of the german language version of the "NCCPC-R"]. Pflege 2007;20(2):93-102. [German]
[43] Breau LM, Gregoire M, Lévêque C, Hennequin M, Bureau N, Wood C. Validation en français de la Grille d'Évaluation de la Douleur-Déficience Intellectuelle. Société Française d'Etude et de Traitement de la Douleur. In press. [French]
[44] Defrin R, Lotan M, Pick CG. The evaluation of acute pain in individuals with cognitive impairment: a differential effect of the level of impairment. Pain 2006;124(3):312-20.
[45] Stephenson JR, Dowrick M. Parent priorities in communication intervention for young students with severe disabilities. Educ Training Ment Retard Dev Disabil 2000;35(1):25-35.
[46] Cassidy KL, Reid GJ, McGrath PJ, Smith DJ, Brown TL, Finley GA. A randomized double-blind, placebo-controlled trial of the EMLA patch for the reduction of pain associated with intramuscular injection in four to six-year-old children. Acta Paediatr 2001; 90(11):1329-36.

[47] Bronfenbrenner U. The ecology of human development: Experiments by nature and design. Cambridge, MA: Harvard Univ Press, 1979.

[48] Breau LM. A bio-ecological approach to pediatric pain assessment. J Pain Managet. In press.

VIII. Maternal Pain and its Long-Term Effects

In: Children and Pain
Editors: P. Schofield and J. Merrick
ISBN 978-1-60876-020-6

Chapter 12

Pregnancy and analgetics: Long term effect on child quality of life

***Søren Ventegodt, MD, MMedSci, EU-MSc**[*1,2,3,4,5]**, Isack Kandel, MA, PhD**[6]**, Patricia Schofield, PhD**[7]**, Efrat Merrick-Kenig, MD**[8]** and Joav Merrick, MD, MMedSci, DMSc**[8,,9,10]*

[1]Quality of Life Research Center, Classensgade 11C,
1 sal, DK-2100 Copenhagen O, Denmark
[2]Research Clinic for Holistic Medicine
[3]Nordic School of Holistic Medicine, Copenhagen, Denmark
[4]Scandinavian Foundation for Holistic Medicine, Sandvika, Norway
[5]Interuniversity College, Graz, Austria
[6]Faculty of Social Sciences, Department of Behavioral Sciences,
Ariel University Center, Samaria, Ariel, Israel
[7]Centre for Advanced Studies in Nursing,
Department of General Practice and Primary Care, University of Aberdeen,
Aberdeen, United Kingdom
[8]National Institute of Child Health and Human Development
[9]Office of the Medical Director, Division for Mental Retardation,
Ministry of Social Affairs, Jerusalem, Israel
[10]Kentucky Children's Hospital,
University of Kentucky, Lexington, United States

Abstract

The objective of this chapter was to explain the global quality of life (QOL) from 2,000 indicators representing all aspects of life. Design and setting was a prospective cohort study with 7,222 members of the Copenhagen Perinatal Birth Cohort 1959-61 (with a 31-

[*] Correspondence: Søren Ventegodt, MD, MMedSci, MSc, Director, Quality of Life Research Center, Classensgade 11C, 1 sal, DK-2100 Copenhagen O, Denmark. Tel: +45-33-141113; Fax: +45-33-141123; E-mail: ventegodt@livskvalitet.org

33 years follow-up) and 9,006 mothers and their 8,820 children born in Copenhagen 1959-1961. Main outcome measures: Global QOL measured by SEQOL (self evaluation of quality of life) containing eight global QOL measures: Well-being, life-satisfaction, happiness, fulfilment of needs, experience of temporal and spatial domains, expression of life's potentials and objective factors. Results: Among 2,000 associations the mother's use of analgesics during pregnancy seems to have a radical and negative impact on the child's quality of life 33 years later. Conclusions: Quality of life is strongly associated with mother's use of analgesics, making this group of drugs highly suspicious for giving serious damage to the fetus. Pregnant women should avoid analgesic drugs and use complementary and alternative medical methods to reduce pain and discomfort. Analgesics during pregnancy should only be available with prescription from a physician.

Introduction

The concept of quality of life (QOL) has become an important topic both in the health field, social welfare and the political debate, especially in the Nordic countries. Enhancing the quality of life is more and more considered to be an objective in treatment and prevention of illness together with the provision of psychosocial support. For the last three decades QOL has been a major issue of debate in Denmark, and in recent years the concept of quality of life or living "a good life" has been the subject of a number of philosophical and psychological studies in Denmark made by other researchers before us (Aggernæs, 1989 (1); Henriksen, 1992 (2); Holm et al, 1994 (3); Kemp, 1991 (4); Sandøe, 1992 (5)). It is becoming increasingly apparent that illness is closely related to the individual perception of a good life, and therefore the exploration of indicators related to quality of life appears to be of broad importance for the prevention and treatment of diseases.

Our search for describing quality of life was built on the foundation that our quality of life must be composed of items that are known to us. Therefore a comparative valuation of these items must be our chief instrument for deciding the degree of quality of life of the person studied. The best quality of life will be the state that contains the greatest number of items having a positive value according to our own estimate. In order to arrive at correct decisions as to which items should be included in the questionnaire, it was necessary to consider what we would judge to be good and consider what comparative values to attach each item. From this approach we created first the SEQOL (self evaluation of quality of life) questionnaire, and later the much shorter and easier-used QOL1 and QOL5 questionnaires.

Identifying, which factors constitute a good life may reveal an understanding about what areas in life should be encouraged, in order to enhance the global quality of life, health, and ability. In this paper we present results from studies initiated in 1989 to examine quality of life in relation to disease. The purpose of this chapter is to assemble the results from the study carried out in the years between 1993 and 1997, examining a total of 11.500 Danes, to show the association between quality of life and a wide series of social indicators, in the ambition to make an almost complete map of QOL and the factors determining QOL, physical and mental health, and sexual, social and working ability (see the published series of papers below). We include three major lines of indicators: indicators of the present life, indicators of the personal history (life events), and indicators from the beginning of life, including a series of social and biological factors. Our belief was that a part of the variation of QOL in the adult population could be explained by biological and social heritage, another part could be explained by life event – happy and unhappy – and a third part could be explained by the conscious choices in life, recently, here and now.

Much to our surprise, data came out back in 1993-5 that convincingly showed us that our human consciousness seems to be the all-dominating factor that determines our quality of life, health, and ability. This discovery lead us to explore the possibilities for interviewing directly on human consciousness, and we found three major sources of knowledge on the intervention on the human consciousness for medical reasons: the classical holistic Hippocratic character medicine which includes conversational therapy, bodywork, and spiritual exercises; the integrative and transcultural medicine that integrates all the medical systems of the pre-mordern cultures which most often also used conversational therapy, bodywork, and spiritual exercises with a major focus on bodywork and spiritual exercises, and the tradition of psychoanalysis and psychodynamic therapy, primarily conversational therapy but in some modern traditions also including bodywork.

In 1997 the Quality of Life Research Center took the initiative to establish an international research team to meet the huge challenge of developing such a contemporary, medical synthesis aiming at integrating all existent consciousness-oriented (holistic) medical knowledge. Around the year 2000 the team had 20 members from three continents working together to create what today is called scientific or clinical, holistic medicine. In 1997 the Research Clinic for Holistic Medicine (CHM) was established, and thanks to substantial funding from the IMK Almene Foundation though all these years – including the four floor building called "The House of Health" that was created in central Copenhagen with funding of about 4 mill. EUROs. Here the new medical synthesis CHM was developed and tested on 500 volunteers most of them with severe, subjective, chronic health problems, which could not be sufficiently helped by biomedicine (drugs or surgery).

To conclude the introduction, Quality of Life Research Center is today a small, private research center, a NGO. It started at the University Hospital in the early 1990s, and became independent in 1994. Its mission is research and development in quality of life, health and ability, and in the development of these crucial factors in life. To succeed with this hardly manageable mission, the center has from its beginning chosen to work in international networks, and in assuming an abstract and holistic approach to health sciences.

The peer-reviewed papers from Quality of Life Research Center has been published in the following series; to understand why so many different interpretations of data are possible we must strongly recommend that the reader gets himself familiar with at least the series 2,3,6, and 12:

1. QOL methodology (6-14) describing how global QOL can be measured.
2. QOL philosophy (15-21) suggesting a holistic way to re-think medical science.
3. QOL theory (22-24) describing different ways to understand QOL scientifically.
4. QOL questionnaires (25,26) is three validated tools to measure global QOL and subjective physical and mental health.
5. QOL results (27-37) is our statistical findings.

6. Theories of existence (38-46) is our speculations on the true nature of the human existence (or wholeness, or “soul”, or conscious roots of being)
7. Holistic medicine (47-50) describes our research programs and methods for documenting effects of holistic healing, and the theory for holistic healing in individual therapy and a group setting.
8. QOL as medicine (51-53) describes three pilot studies.
9. Clinical holistic medicine (54-90) describes our new synthesis of Hippocratic, transcultural and psychodynamic approaches to consciousness-based medicine.
10. CHM: clinical results (91-96) is the first promising results from the clinical testing of scientific holistic medicine
11. Antonovsky and the sense of coherence (97-102) are six important papers testing the connection between sense of coherence and health.
12. Human Development (103-112) is a new series of papers going into a deeper exploration of the nature of reality, trying to understand biological information and the connection between matter, life and consciousness.

What we did

To explore the association between quality of life and the various different indicators, it was necessary to create a questionnaire that could describe the quality of life of the persons studied (7-14,25,26).

After preliminary background literature research that examined various methods of measuring the quality of life, a study group on “quality-of-life research” was established in Copenhagen in order to investigate the field and identify a number of theories on the subject (22-24). A subgroup was formed to construct a questionnaire with the purpose of investigating the quality of life empirically within selected cohorts. During 1991-1993, this questionnaire was revised and improved in twenty pilot studies through qualitative interviews. In addition, a number of pilot surveys on different groups refined the questionnaire further. We found it ready for use in its present form in 1993.

All four studies are based on the same SEQOL questionnaire (Self Evaluation of Quality of Life questionnaire) (25,26), which measures the global quality of life. The questionnaire consists of 317 items and based on an “integrative” theory of the quality of life, a theoretical framework from a Danish QOL survey involving 7,222 persons 31-33 year olds (see figure 1), measuring it across eight different global QOL dimensions (22).

The integrative QOL theory was created to organize a number of theories on the quality of life into a spectrum that spans the extremes of subjective and objective quality of life. SEQOL is a self-administered questionnaires with items rated on five-point Likert scales. For validation SEQOL was send to 2,460 persons 18-88 year olds randomly selected from the Danish Central Person Register (CPR-Register) together with the Nottingham Health profile (NHP), Sickness Impact Factor (SIP), and the test-retest reliability correlation was >0.8, Cronbach’s alpha was 0.75, correlation (r) to NHP was 0,49, to SIP 0.27 ($P<0.05$). Adjustment for health status made the correlation to SIP stronger among the sick ($r=0.41$). For SEQOL 111 respondents were needed to detect 3% difference in QOL. SEQOL is thus valid as it shows a high level of reliability, sensitivity and consistency. For the calculation of the global QOL, 113 of the questions are used. The rest is control questions and questions giving more information about health status, sexuality, philosophy of life, life style, self-perception, and social circumstances. The principle of SEQOL is that of a hierarchy of factors, adding up to an abstract total QOL. These measures are showed below (sample questions from the questionnaire included):

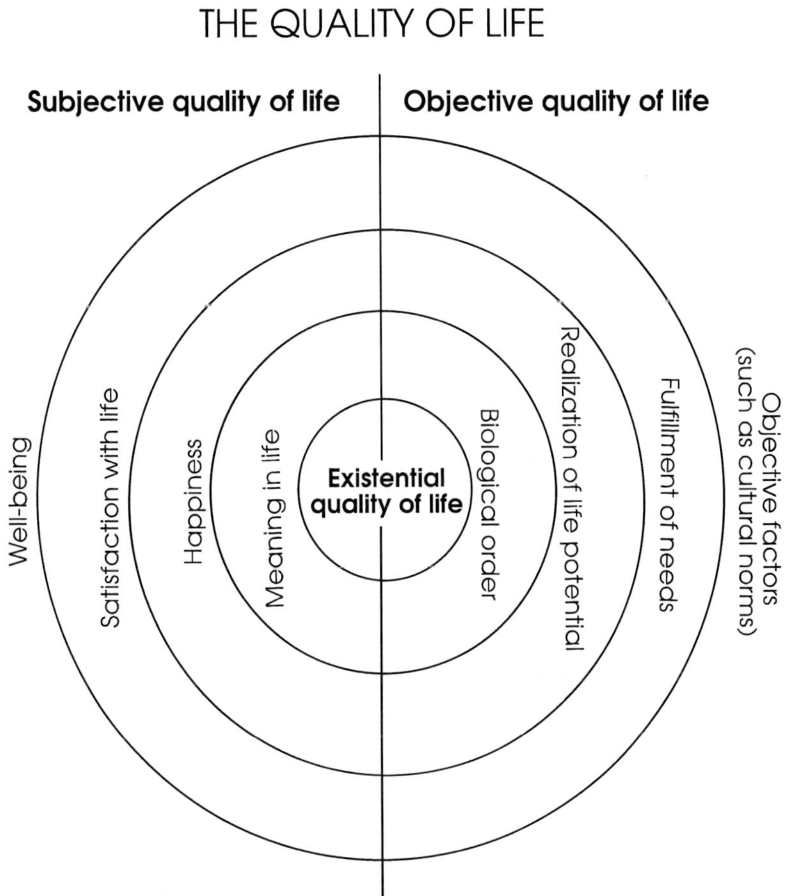

Figure 1. The integrative (IQOL) theory of the quality of life. The individual can best be compared to a green apple with red patches (a subjective and an objective quality of life, respectively at the surface of an individual's existence) with a hidden nucleus (humanity's inner depth). When this picture is combined with the picture of humanity as an onion with a number of layers between the surface and the nucleus, the taxonomy underlying the quality-of-life analysis is achieved. Between life's surface and its inexpressible depth lies well-being, satisfaction, harmony and meaning and deep concord (22).

Subjective measures

1. Immediate, self-experienced well-being ("How are you feeling?")
2. Life satisfaction ("How satisfying is your life?")

3. Happiness ("How happy are you at present?")

Existential measures

4. Fulfilment of needs (e.g., "How well are your social needs ful¬filled?")
5. Experience of life's temporal domains (e.g., "How do you feel when you are at home?")
6. Experience of life's spatial domains ("How satisfied are you with [each of five domains: self, partner, family, friends, community]")
7. Expression of life's potentials [to which extent are they fulfilled]

Objective measure

8. Objective factors [income, status, work etc.]

Replies to each of the questions that constitute these measures were weighted and scored to yield computable numbers between a minimum of 0 and a maximum of 100 (7-14), for all technical details see also (113-117). These numbers are then taken as representing the quality of life of the re¬spondent, expressed in terms of the eight different ways the quality of life has been measured by the questionnaire. Suitably weighted and scored, replies to the first part of the questionnaire constitute variables, the co-variation of which the quality of life can be calculated.

Measuring quality of life has been the subject for many disagreements through time. In our research, the global QOL - in the most broad and all-including sense - is the primary outcome measure (dependent variable); the integrative QOL theory made us include 113 items in SEQOL questionnaire for the calculation of the global QOL (117)).

In this study we had to deal with an essential problem: When the statistical connection between 113 life factors and the global QOL was measured, we often had a contribution to the statistical co-variation from the construction of the global QOL measure. Lets give an example: The objective QOL measure (no. 8) includes a question on having a partner or not:

Do you have a partner?

1 Yes
2 In doubt
3 No

If a person says yes, and we want to analyse the statistical connection with marital status and global QOL, we will get a contribution from the way the objective QOL is defined and measured because having a partner gives a likelihood for being married.

This problem turned out to be of little significance, as even the most strongly "constructed" connections did not count for more that 1/15th of the total connection. Still this gives an error of up to 7% in co-variation, for which we have compensated in a further analysis.

As the large connections in our study showed a co-variation of 20% global QOL or more, the above-mentioned error introduced by the construction of the global all-including QOL measure is generally neglectable. It is important to notice that the way our QOL measure was constructed this does not constitute a measuring problem; we will almost always find a high correlation when N=5-10.000 between QOL and the many factors constituting the global QOL or the factors related to them. However, we are not looking at the size of the correlation (the statistical significance), but at the size of the statistical co-variation (QOL difference in %) showing the clinical significance (9).

The study is a prospective cohort study investigating the connection between quality of life and a thousand early life factors (6-37,113-116). The cohort included 7,222 persons from the Copenhagen Perinatal Birth Cohort and the results showed the connection between an early life factor and the quality of life of the child 31-33 years later. In the studies including a total of 7700 Danes, we have about 2,000 factors correlated to the global QOL.

Examples from the SEQOL questionnaire are

Q14. With whom do you live?

1 living alone
2 spouse or partner
3 own children
4 partners children
5 adopted children
6 friends
7 biological parents
8 others.

Q127. How satisfied are you with your sex life now?

1 very satisfied
2 satisfied
3 neither satisfied nor dissatisfied
4 dissatisfied
5 very dissatisfied

We have found "satisfaction with your sex life (men) 30.9%", meaning that the difference between best category (very satisfied, 11.1% above the average) and worst category (very unsatisfied, 19.8% below average) showed a difference of 30.9%. Here we have a continuous variable making it more meaningful and exact to analyse the co-variation using (modified) linear regression (6-14). Using these different ways of analysing the size of the co-variation makes it possible to compare the co-variation of the different life factors with respect to the global QOL.

The size of the co-variation gives us the clinical significans, which is impossible to judge from the statistical correlation alone (the statistical significanse). We have invented a method to obtain a direct quantitative measure of the statistical co-variation, making it possible to compare all the associations directly and quantitatively, instead of using the Cohen's suggestion of simply interpreting effect size as "low", "medium" and "high".

Our findings

We found a strong association between quality of life and mothers use of analgesics during pregnancy; we also found all other drugs – except the psychopharmacological drugs - did not show this association. If mother used analgesics in the during the first month of pregnancy, we found that the child's total integrative quality of life (I-QOL)(22) was 59.4% or 10.6% below average of 70.0%; life satisfaction and happiness is also significantly lover ($P<0.05\%$). If mother used analgesics in 2nd month of pregnancy the child was 9.3% below average, and if she used them in third month of pregnancy, the child was 6.9% lover in I-QOL 33 years later. These findings are highly significant ($p<0.01$). If mother used analgesics in the 2nd trimester, the child was 3.3% below average in I-QOL ($p<0.05$). If mother used analgesics in the in 3rd trimester the children's quality of life is 4.0% lower ($p<0.01$). Using analgesics the last month of pregnancy is association with an I-QOL 4.2% lover than average ($p<0.05$). Even just using painkillers once during pregnancy was associated with an I-QOL 0.9% below average, which indicates that there were serious reasons to recommend complete abstinence from painkillers during pregnancy! No other drugs on the long list recorded by the researchers in 1959-61 were associated with a similar lowering of the quality of life (Antihistamines, anti-epileptics, Barbiturates, psychopharmacological drugs i.e. largactil and meprobamate), antibiotics, chemotherapy, hormones, anti-hormones, diuretics, other drugs). A smaller association was found between using psychopharmacological drugs and child's QOL 31-33 years later; these data will be presented in an other paper.

Discussion

The Danish Quality of Life Survey is based on the Danish Perinatal Birth Cohort 1959-61, which consisted of 9,008 mothers and their children that we have followed over time. As such birth cohorts are extremely rare, because they are expensive and time-consuming to conduct, and since long-term follow-up of the global QOL is a recent idea, we have to our knowledge not seen similar studies carried out in the world. We therefore believe our data and findings to be of a unique nature. For a more general approuach to QOL we refer to the database on happiness by Ruut Veenhoven 2004 (http://worlddatabaseofhappiness.eur.nl). Other studies have similar designs as the present study, but are focused on health-related QOL, behavior, self confidence or life-satisfaction, and not global QOL.

Table 1. Presents the impact on child's QOL from Analgesic

	Immediate self-experienced well-being		Life satisfaction		Happiness		Fullfilment of needs		Experience of objective tempora domains		Experience of objective spatial domains		Expression of life's potentials		Objective factors		Test (p-value)	Total IQOL
	%	n	%	n	%	n	%	n	%	n	%	n	%	n	%	n		%
First month	59,6	23	57,0	23	55,2	23	61,6	19	63,0	22	59,1	23	50,0	23	62,5	21	0.0002**	59,4
Second month	62,3	26	60,8	26	56,9	26	62,5	22	66,0	25	61,2	26	50,2	26	62,2	24	0.0004**	60,7
Third month	62,4	34	61,2	34	59,4	34	63,3	29	69,2	33	62,2	34	52,4	34	66,6	32	0.0034**	63,1
2 trimester	70,0	74	68,4	74	64,6	74	65,9	63	72,6	71	63,9	70	56,6	74	67,7	69	0.0297*	66,7
3 trimester	69,0	81	64,8	81	62,9	79	66,1	73	70,6	77	64,1	81	58,1	79	67,7	78	0.0058**	66,0
Last month	69,4	72	66,4	72	64,3	70	66,9	66	70,6	69	63,4	71	57,4	70	66,2	68	0.0125*	65,8
One time	71,1	157	68,0	157	65,5	155	66,5	142	72,6	152	65,0	152	58,1	155	69,6	150	0.0267*	67,8
None	72,0	2105	69,4	2106	66,1	2106	68,4	1929	74,9	2080	67,2	2048	61,8	2096	72,8	2060	0.4982	70,0

The data presented in this paper suggested that the child was extremely vulnerable to mother's use of painkillers during pregnancy, with the most damage happening to the fetus in the first trimester. This is most unfortunately, as a woman with an active sexual life can never be sure that she is not getting pregnant; and the child could be damaged even before she notices the pregnancy.

There is another possible explanation, and that is that it is the mother having pain itself, so strong that it inspires to using painkillers, that damage the child's QOL and happiness later. But as this is a guess, which cannot be examined in the data, we find it better to try to prevent systematic damage on millions of children by giving this warning now.

The reason for the strongly negative effect on the grown up child's QOL from mothers use of analgesics is most likely to be a direct biological effect of the drug on the foetus. Another possibility is that the negative impact of implanted philosophy from the biomedical treatment (118,119).

Conclusions

The data suggested a strong, negative influence on the child's permanent quality of life, if the mother used painkillers (analgesics) during pregnancy. As the damage seemed to be largest in the beginning of pregnancy, we must advice all women with an active sex-life to abstain from using painkillers, unless this is absolutely necessary. Painkillers should only be allowed with prescription in order to prevent severe damage on the children's quality of life. Further research must be done to establish the exact mechanism that connects use of drug-killers to lower quality of life in the adult children.

Acknowledgements

The Danish Quality of Life Survey and the Quality of Life Research Center was 1991-2004 supported by grants from the 1991 Pharmacy Foundation, the Goodwill-fonden, the JL-Foundation, E Danielsen and Wife's Foundation, Emmerick Meyer's Trust, the Frimodt-Heineken Foundation, the Hede Nielsen Family Foundation, Petrus Andersens Fond, Wholesaler C.P. Frederiksens Study Trust, Else and Mogens Wedell-Wedellsborg's Foundation and IMK Almene Fond. The research was approved by the Copenhagen Scientific Ethical Committee under number (KF)V.100.2123/91 and later correspondance.

References

[1] Aggernæs A. [Quality of life]. Copenhagen: FADL's Publ, 1989. [Danish]
[2] Henriksen BL. [Quality of life]. Copenhagen: Gad, 1992. [Danish]
[3] Holm P, Holst J, Olsen SB, Perlt B. [Life and quality in care and pedagogy]. Herning: Systime, 1994. [Danish]
[4] Kemp P. [The un-replacable]. Copenhagen: Spektrum, 1991. [Danish]

[5] Sandøe P. [Quality of life and ethics]. Copenhagen: Nyt Nordisk Forlag Arnold Busck, 1992. [Danish]
[6] Ventegodt S, Flensborg-Madsen T, Andersen NJ, Nielsen M, Mohammed M, Merrick J. Global quality of life (QOL), health and ability are primarily determined by our consciousness. Research findings from Denmark 1991-2004. Soc Indicator Res 2005;71:87-122.
[7] Ventegodt S, Merrick J, Andersen NJ. A new method for generic measuring of the global quality of life. ScientificWorldJournal 2003;3:946-9.
[8] Ventegodt S, Hilden J, Merrick J. Measurement of quality of life I: A methodological framework. ScientificWorldJournal 2003;3:950-61.
[9] Ventegodt S, Merrick J, Andersen NJ. Measurement of quality of life II. From philosophy of life to science. ScientificWorldJournal 2003;3:962-71.
[10] Ventegodt S, Merrick J, Andersen NJ. Measurement of quality of life III: From the IQOL theory to the global, generic SEQOL questionnaire. ScientificWorldJournal 2003;3:972-91.
[11] Ventegodt S, Merrick J, Andersen NJ. Measurement of quality of life IV: Use of the SEQOL, QOL5, QOL1 and other global and generic questionnaires. ScientificWorldJournal 2003;3:992-1001.
[12] Ventegodt S, Merrick J, Andersen NJ. Measurement of quality of life V: How to use the SEQOL, QOL5, QOL1 and other and generic questionnaires for research. ScientificWorldJournal 2003;3:1002-14.
[13] Ventegodt S, Merrick J, Andersen NJ. Measurement of quality of life VI: Quality-adjusted life years (QALY) is an unfortunate use of quality of life concept. ScientificWorldJournal 2003;3:1015-9.
[14] Ventegodt S, Merrick J. Measurement of quality of life VII: Statistical covariation and global quality of life data. The method of weight-modified linear regression. ScientificWorldJournal 2003;3:1020-9.
[15] Ventegodt S, Andersen NJ, Merrick J. Quality of life philosophy: when life sparkles or can we make wisdom a science? ScientificWorldJournal 2003;3:1160-3.
[16] Ventegodt S, Andersen NJ, Merrick J. QOL philosophy I: Quality of life, happiness, and meaning of life. ScientificWorldJournal 2003;3:1164-75.
[17] Ventegodt S, Andersen NJ, Kromann M, Merrick J. QOL philosophy II: What is a human being? ScientificWorldJournal 2003;3:1176-85.
[18] Ventegodt S, Merrick J, Andersen NJ. QOL philosophy III: Towards a new biology. ScientificWorldJournal 2003;3:1186-98.
[19] Ventegodt S, Andersen NJ, Merrick J. QOL philosophy IV: The brain and consciousness. ScientificWorldJournal 2003;3:1199-1209.
[20] Ventegodt S, Andersen NJ, Merrick J. QOL philosophy V: Seizing the meaning of life and getting well again. ScientificWorldJournal 2003;3:1210-29.
[21] Ventegodt S, Andersen NJ, Merrick J. QOL philosophy VI: The concepts. ScientificWorldJournal 2003;3:1230-40.
[22] Ventegodt S, Merrick J, Andersen NJ. Quality of life theory I. The IQOL theory: An integrative theory of the global quality of life concept. ScientificWorldJournal 2003;3:1030-40.
[23] Ventegodt S, Merrick J, Andersen NJ. Quality of life theory II. Quality of life as the realization of life potential: A biological theory of human being. ScientificWorldJournal 2003;3:1041-9.
[24] Ventegodt S, Merrick J, Andersen NJ. Quality of life theory III. Maslow revisited. ScientificWorldJournal 2003;3:1050-7.
[25] Ventegodt S, Henneberg EW, Merrick J, Lindholt JS. Validation of two global and generic quality of life questionnaires for population screening: SCREENQOL and SEQOL. ScientificWorldJournal 2003;3:412-21.
[26] Lindholt JS, Ventegodt S, Henneberg EW. Development and validation of QoL5 for clinical databases. A short, global and generic questionnaire based on an integrated theory of the quality of life. Eur J Surg 2002;168:103-7.
[27] Ventegodt S. Sex and the quality of life in Denmark. Arch Sex Behav 1998;27(3):295-307.
[28] Ventegodt S. A prospective study on quality of life and traumatic events in early life – 30 year follow-up. Child Care Health Dev 1998;25(3):213-21.

[29] Ventegodt S, Merrick J. Long-term effects of maternal smoking on quality of life. Results from the Copenhagen Perinatal Birth Cohort 1959-61. ScientificWorld Journal 2003;3:714-20.

[30] Ventegodt S, Merrick J. Long-term effects of maternal medication on global quality of life measured with SEQOL. Results from the Copenhagen Perinatal Birth Cohort 1959-61. ScientificWorldJournal 2003;3:707-13.

[31] Ventegodt S, Merrick J. Psychoactive drugs and quality of life. ScientificWorldJournal 2003;3:694-706.

[32] Ventegodt S, Merrick J. Lifestyle, quality of life and health. ScientificWorldJournal 2003;3:811-25.

[33] Ventegodt S, Flensborg-Madsen T, Andersen NJ, Merrick J. The health and social situation of the mother during pregnancy and global quality of life of the child as an adult. Results from the prospective Copenhagen Perinatal Cohort 1959-1961. ScientificWorldJournal 2005;5:950-8.

[34] Ventegodt S, Flensborg-Madsen T, Anderson NJ, Merrick J. Factors during pregnancy, delivery and birth affecting global quality of life of the adult child at long-term follow-up. Results from the prospective Copenhagen Perinatal Birth Cohort 1959-61. ScientificWorldJournal 2005;5:933-41.

[35] Ventegodt S, Flensborg-Madsen T, Andersen NJ, Merrick J. Events in pregnancy, delivery, and infancy and long-term effects on global quality of life: results from the Copenhagen Perinatal Birth Cohort 1959-61. Med Sci Monit 2005;11(8):CR357-65.

[36] Ventegodt S, Flensborg-Madsen T, Andersen NJ, Morad M, Merrick J. Quality of life and events in the first year of life. Results from the prospective Copenhagen Birth Cohort 1959-61. ScientificWorldJournal 2006;6:106-15.

[37] Ventegodt S, Flensborg-Madsen T, Andersen NJ, Merrick J. What influence do major events in life have on our later quality of life? A retrospective study on life events and associated emotions. Med Sci Monit 2006;12(2):SR9-15.

[38] Ventegodt S, Andersen NJ, Merrick J. Five theories of human existence. ScientificWorldJournal 2003;3:1272-6.

[39] Ventegodt S. The life mission theory: A theory for a consciousness-based medicine. Int J Adolesc Med Health 2003;15(1): 89-91.

[40] Ventegodt S, Andersen NJ, Merrick J. The life mission theory II: The structure of the life purpose and the ego. ScientificWorldJournal 2003;3:1277-85.

[41] Ventegodt S, Andersen NJ, Merrick J. The life mission theory III: Theory of talent. ScientificWorldJournal 2003;3:1286-93.

[42] Ventegodt S, Merrick J. The life mission theory IV. A theory of child development. ScientificWorldJournal 2003;3:1294-1301.

[43] Ventegodt S, Andersen NJ, Merrick J. The life mission theory V. A theory of the anti-self and explaining the evil side of man. ScientificWorldJournal 2003;3:1302-13.

[44] Ventegodt S, Andersen NJ, Merrick J. The life mission theory VI: A theory for the human character. ScientificWorldJournal 2004;4:859-80.

[45] Ventegodt S, Flensborg-Madsen T, Andersen NJ, Merrick J. Life mission theory VII: Theory of existential (Antonovsky) coherence: a theory of quality of life, health and ability for use in holistic medicine. ScientificWorldJournal 2005;5:377-89.

[46] Ventegodt S, Kandel I, Merrick J. Life mission theory VIII: A theory for pain. J Pain Manage 2008;1(1):5-10.

[47] Ventegodt S, Andersen NJ, Merrick J. Holistic medicine: Scientific challenges. ScientificWorldJournal 2003;3:1108-16.

[48] Ventegodt S, Andersen NJ, Merrick J. Holistic Medicine II: The square-curve paradigm for research in alternative, complementary and holistic medicine: A cost-effective, easy and scientifically valid design for evidence based medicine. ScientificWorldJournal 2003;3: 1117-27.

[49] Ventegodt S, Andersen NJ, Merrick J. Holistic Medicine III: The holistic process theory of healing. ScientificWorldJournal 2003;3:1138-46.

[50] Ventegodt S, Andersen NJ, Merrick J. Holistic Medicine IV: Principles of the holistic process of healing in a group setting. ScientificWorldJournal 2003;3:1294-1301.
[51] Ventegodt S, Andersen NJ, Merrick J. Quality of life as medicine. A pilot study of patients with chronic illness and pain. ScientificWorldJournal 2003;3:520-32.
[52] Ventegodt S, Andersen NJ, Merrick J. Quality of life as medicine II. A pilot study of a five-day "Quality of Life and Health" cure for patients with alcoholism. ScientificWorldJournal 2003;3:842-52.
[53] Ventegodt S, Clausen B, Langhorn M, Kroman M, Andersen NJ, Merrick J. Quality of life as medicine III. A qualitative analysis of the effect of a five days intervention with existential holistic group therapy or a quality of life course as a modern rite of passage. ScientificWorldJournal 2004;4:124-33.
[54] Ventegodt S. Every contact with the patient must be therapeutic. J Pediatr Adolesc Gynecol 2007;20(6):323-4.
[55] Ventegodt S, Merrick J. Psychosomatic reasons for chronic pains. South Med J 2005;98(11):1063.
[56] Ventegodt S, Merrick J. Clinical holistic medicine: Applied consciousness-based medicine. ScientificWorldJournal 2004;4:96-9.
[57] Ventegodt S, Morad M, Merrick J. Clinical holistic medicine: Classic art of healing or the therapeutic touch. ScientificWorldJournal 2004;4:134-47.
[58] Ventegodt S, Morad M, Merrick J. Clinical holistic medicine: The "new medicine", the multi-paradigmatic physician and the medical record. ScientificWorldJournal 2004;4:273-85.
[59] Ventegodt S, Morad M, Merrick J. Clinical holistic medicine: Holistic pelvic examination and holistic treatment of infertility. ScientificWorldJournal 2004;4:148-58.
[60] Ventegodt S, Morad M, Hyam E, Merrick J. Clinical holistic medicine: Use and limitations of the biomedical paradigm ScientificWorldJournal 2004;4:295-306.
[61] Ventegodt S, Morad M, Kandel I, Merrick J. Clinical holistic medicine: Social problems disguised as illness. ScientificWorldJournal 2004;4:286-94.
[62] Ventegodt S, Morad M, Andersen NJ, Merrick J. Clinical holistic medicine Tools for a medical science based on consciousness. ScientificWorldJournal 2004;4:347-61.
[63] Ventegodt S, Morad M, Merrick J. Clinical holistic medicine: Prevention through healthy lifestyle and quality of life. Oral Health Prev Dent 2004;1:239-45.
[64] Ventegodt S, Morad M, Hyam E, Merrick J. Clinical holistic medicine: When biomedicine is inadequate. ScientificWorldJournal 2004;4:333-46.
[65] Ventegodt S, Morad M, Merrick J. Clinical holistic medicine: Holistic treatment of children. ScientificWorldJournal 2004;4:581-8.
[66] Ventegodt S, Morad M, Merrick J. Clinical holistic medicine: Problems in sex and living together. ScientificWorldJournal 2004;4:562-70.
[67] Ventegodt S, Morad M, Hyam E, Merrick J. Clinical holistic medicine: Holistic sexology and treatment of vulvodynia through existential therapy and acceptance through touch. ScientificWorldJournal 2004;4:571-80.
[68] Ventegodt S, Flensborg-Madsen T, Andersen NJ, Morad M, Merrick J. Clinical holistic medicine: A Pilot on HIV and Quality of Life and a Suggested treatment of HIV and AIDS. ScientificWorldJournal 2004;4:264-72.
[69] Ventegodt S, Morad M, Merrick J. Clinical holistic medicine: Induction of spontaneous remission of cancer by recovery of the human character and the purpose of life (the fife mission). ScientificWorldJournal 2004;4:362-77.
[70] Ventegodt S, Morad M, Kandel I, Merrick J. Clinical holistic medicine: Treatment of physical health problems without a known cause, exemplified by hypertension and tinnitus. ScientificWorldJournal 2004;4:716-24.
[71] Ventegodt S, Morad M, Merrick J. Clinical holistic medicine: Developing from asthma, allergy and eczema. ScientificWorldJournal 2004;4:936-42.

[72] Ventegodt S, Morad M, Press J, Merrick J, Shek D. Clinical holistic medicine: Holistic adolescent medicine. ScientificWorldJournal 2004;4:551-61.
[73] Ventegodt S, Solheim E, Saunte ME, Morad M, Kandel I, Merrick J. Clinical holistic medicine: Metastatic cancer. ScientificWorldJournal 2004;4:913-35.
[74] Ventegodt S, Morad M, Kandel I, Merrick J. Clinical holistic medicine: a psychological theory of dependency to improve quality of life. ScientificWorldJournal 2004;4:638-48.
[75] Ventegodt S, Merrick J. Clinical holistic medicine: Chronic infections and autoimmune diseases. ScientificWorldJournal 2005;5: 155-64.
[76] Ventegodt S, Kandel I, Neikrug S, Merrick J. Clinical holistic medicine: Holistic treatment of rape and incest traumas. ScientificWorldJournal 2005;5:288-97.
[77] Ventegodt S, Morad M, Merrick J. Clinical holistic medicine: Chronic pain in the locomotor system. ScientificWorldJournal 2005;5:165-72.
[78] Ventegodt S, Merrick J. Clinical holistic medicine: Chronic pain in internal organs. ScientificWorldJournal 2005;5:205-10.
[79] Ventegodt S, Kandel I, Neikrug S, Merrick J. Clinical holistic medicine: The existential crisis – life crisis, stress and burnout. ScientificWorldJournal 2005;5:300-12.
[80] Ventegodt S, Gringols G, Merrick J. Clinical holistic medicine: Holistic rehabilitation. ScientificWorldJournal 2005;5:280-7.
[81] Ventegodt S, Andersen NJ, Neikrug S, Kandel I, Merrick J. Clinical holistic medicine: Mental disorders in a holistic perspective. ScientificWorldJournal 2005;5:313-23.
[82] Ventegodt S, Andersen NJ, Neikrug S, Kandel I, Merrick J. Clinical holistic medicine: Holistic treatment of mental disorders. ScientificWorldJournal 2005;5:427-45.
[83] Ventegodt S, Merrick J. Clinical holistic medicine: The patient with multiple diseases. ScientificWorldJournal 2005;5:324-39.
[84] Ventegodt S, Clausen B, Nielsen ML, Merrick J. Advanced tools for holistic medicine. ScientificWorldJournal 2006;6:2048-65.
[85] Ventegodt S, Clausen B, Merrick J. Clinical holistic medicine: The case story of Anna: I. Long term effect of child sexual abuse and incest with a treatment approach. ScientificWorldJournal 2006;6:1965-76.
[86] Ventegodt S, Morad M, Merrick J. Clinical holistic medicine: the case story of Anna. II. Patient diary as a tool in treatment. ScientificWorldJournal 2006;6:2006-34.
[87] Ventegodt S, Clausen B, Merrick J. Clinical holistic medicine: The case story of Anna. III. Rehabilitation of philosophy of life during holistic existential therapy for childhood sexual abuse. ScientificWorldJournal 2006;6:2080-91.
[88] Ventegodt S, Merrick J. Suicide from a holistic point of view. ScientificWorldJournal. 2005;5:759-66.
[89] Ventegodt S, Clausen B, Omar HA, Merrick J. Clinical holistic medicine: Holistic sexology and acupressure through the vagina (Hippocratic pelvic massage). ScientificWorldJournal 2006;6:2066-79.
[90] Ventegodt S, Clausen B, Merrick J. Clinical holistic medicine: Pilot study on the effect of vaginal acupressure (Hippocratic pelvic massage). ScientificWorldJournal 2006;6:2100-16.
[91] Ventegodt S, Thegler S, Andreasen T, Struve F, Enevoldsen L, Bassaine L, Torp M, Merrick J. Clinical holistic medicine: Psychodynamic short-time therapy complemented with bodywork. A clinical follow-up study of 109 Patients. ScientificWorldJournal 2006;6:2220-38.
[92] Ventegodt S, Thegler S, Andreasen T, Struve F, Enevoldsen L, Bassaine L, Torp M, Merrick J. Clinical holistic medicine (mindful, short-term psychodynamic psychotherapy complemented with bodywork) in the treatment of experienced impaired sexual functioning. ScientificWorldJournal 2007;7:324-9.
[93] Ventegodt S, Thegler S, Andreasen T, Struve F, Enevoldsen L, Bassaine L, Torp M, Merrick J. Clinical holistic medicine (mindful, short-term psychodynamic psychotherapy complemented with

bodywork) improves quality of life, health, and ability by induction of Antonovsky-salutogenesis. ScientificWorldJournal 2007;7:317-23.
[94] Ventegodt S, Thegler S, Andreasen T, Struve F, Enevoldsen L, Bassaine L, Torp M, Merrick J. Clinical holistic medicine (mindful, short-term psychodynamic psychotherapy complemented with bodywork) in the treatment of experienced physical illness and chronic pain. ScientificWorldJournal 2007;7:310-6
[95] Ventegodt S, Thegler S, Andreasen T, Struve F, Enevoldsen L, Bassaine L, Torp M, Merrick J. Clinical holistic medicine (mindful, short-term psychodynamic psychotherapy complemented with bodywork) in the treatment of experienced mental illness. ScientificWorldJournal 2007;7:306-9.
[96] Ventegodt S, Thegler S, Andreasen T, Struve F, Enevoldsen L, Bassaine L, Torp M, Merrick J. Self-reported low self-esteem. Intervention and follow-up in a clinical setting. ScientificWorldJournal 2007;7:299-305.
[97] Flensborg-Madsen T, Ventegodt S, Merrick J. Sense of coherence and physical health. A Review of previous findings. ScientificWorldJournal 2005;5:665-73.
[98] Flensborg-Madsen T, Ventegodt S, Merrick J. Why is Antonovsky's sense of coherence not correlated to physical health? Analysing Antonovsky's 29-item sense of coherence scale (SOCS). ScientificWorldJournal 2005;5:767-76.
[99] Flensborg-Madsen T, Ventegodt S, Merrick J. Sense of coherence and health. The construction of an amendment to Antonovsky's sense of coherence scale (SOC II). ScientificWorldJournal 2006;6:2133-9.
[100] Flensborg-Madsen T, Ventegodt S, Merrick J. Sense of coherence and physical health. A cross-sectional study using a new SOC scale (SOC II). ScientificWorldJournal 2006;6:2200-11.
[101] Flensborg-Madsen T, Ventegodt S, Merrick J. Sense of coherence and physical health. Testing Antonovsky's theory. ScientificWorldJournal 2006;6:2212-9.
[102] Flensborg-Madsen T, Ventegodt S, Merrick J. Sense of coherence and health. The emotional sense of coherence (SOC-E) was found to be the best-known predictor of physical health. ScientificWorldJournal 2006;6:2147-57.
[103] Hermansen TD, Ventegodt S, Rald E, Clausen B, Nielsen ML, Merrick J. Human development I: twenty fundamental problems of biology, medicine, and neuro-psychology related to biological information. ScientificWorldJournal 2006;6:747-59.
[104] Ventegodt S, Hermansen TD, Nielsen ML, Clausen B, Merrick J. Human development II: we need an integrated theory for matter, life and consciousness to understand life and healing. ScientificWorldJournal 2006;6:760-6.
[105] Ventegodt S, Hermansen TD, Rald E, Flensborg-Madsen T, Nielsen ML, Clausen B, Merrick J. Human development III: bridging brain-mind and body-mind. introduction to "deep" (fractal, poly-ray) cosmology. ScientificWorldJournal 2006;6:767-76.
[106] Ventegodt S, Hermansen TD, Flensborg-Madsen T, Nielsen ML, Clausen B, Merrick J. Human development IV: the living cell has information-directed self-organisation. ScientificWorldJournal 2006;6:1132-8.
[107] Ventegodt S, Hermansen TD, Flensborg-Madsen T, Nielsen ML, Clausen B, Merrick J. Human development V: biochemistry unable to explain the emergence of biological form (morphogenesis) and therefore a new principle as source of biological information is needed. ScientificWorldJournal 2006;6:1359-67.
[108] Ventegodt S, Hermansen TD, Flensborg-Madsen T, Nielsen M, Merrick J. Human development VI: Supracellular morphogenesis. The origin of biological and cellular order. ScientificWorldJournal 2006;6:1424-33.
[109] Ventegodt S, Hermansen TD, Flensborg-Madsen T, Rald E, Nielsen ML, Merrick J. Human development VII: A spiral fractal model of fine structure of physical energy could explain central aspects of biological information, biological organization and biological creativity. ScientificWorldJournal 2006;6:1434-40.

[110] Ventegodt S, Hermansen TD, Flensborg-Madsen T, Nielsen ML, Merrick J. Human development VIII: A theory of "deep" quantum chemistry and cell consciousness: Quantum chemistry controls genes and biochemistry to give cells and higher organisms consciousness and complex behavior. ScientificWorldJournal 2006;6:1441-53.

[111] Ventegodt S, Hermansen TD, Flensborg-Madsen T, Rald E, Nielsen ML, Merrick J. Human development IX: A model of the wholeness of man, his consciousness and collective consciousness. ScientificWorldJournal 2006;6:1454-9.

[112] Hermansen TD, Ventegodt S, Merrick J. Human development X: Explanation of macroevolution — top-down evolution materializes consciousness. The origin of metamorphosis. ScientificWorldJournal 2006;6:1656-66.

[113] Ventegodt S. Quality of life in Denmark. Results from a population survey. Copenhagen: Forskningscentrets Forlag, 1995. [Danish]

[114] Ventegodt S. The Quality of Life of 4500 31-33 year-olds. Result from a study of the Prospective Pediatric Cohort of persons born at the University Hospital in Copenhagen. Copenhagen: Forskningscentrets Forlag, 1996. [Danish]

[115] Ventegodt S. The quality of life and factors in pregnancy, birth and infancy. Results from a follow-up study of the Prospective Pediatric Cohort of persons born at the University Hospital in Copenhagen 1959-61. Copenhagen: Forskningscentrets Forlag, 1995. [Danish]

[116] Ventegodt S. The quality of life and major events in life. Copenhagen: Forskningscentrets Forlag, 2000. [Danish]

[117] Ventegodt S. Measuring the quality of life. From theory to practice. Copenhagen: Forskningscentrets Forlag, 1996.

[118] Ventegodt S, Kandel I, Merrick J. Clinical holistic medicine: How to recover memory without "implanting" memories in your patient. ScientificWorldJournal 2007;7:1579–89.

[119] Ventegodt S, Kandel I, Merrick J. A study of experienced chronic pain in the holistic medicine clinic using mindful short-term psychodynamic psychoterapy complemented with bodywork. J Pain Manage 2008;1(1):55-62.

In: Children and Pain
Editors: P. Schofield and J. Merrick

ISBN 978-1-60876-020-6

Chapter 13

Pregnancy and mental pain: Long term effect of maternal psychopharmacological drugs during pregnancy on child quality of life

Søren Ventegodt, MD, MMedSci, EU-MSc*[*1,2,3,4,5], Efrat Merrick-Kenig, MD[6] and Joav Merrick, MD, MMedSci, DMSc[6,7,8]

[1]Quality of Life Research Center, Classensgade 11C, 1 sal, DK-2100 Copenhagen O, Denmark
[2]Research Clinic for Holistic Medicine
[3]Nordic School of Holistic Medicine, Copenhagen, Denmark
[4]Scandinavian Foundation for Holistic Medicine, Sandvika, Norway
[5]Interuniversity College, Graz, Austria
[6]National Institute of Child Health and Human Development
[7]Office of the Medical Director, Division for Mental Retardation, Ministry of Social Affairs, Jerusalem, Israel
[8]Kentucky Children's Hospital, University of Kentucky, Lexington, United States

Abstract

This chapter will examine the association between maternal use of psychopharmacologic drugs during pregnancy and the child's quality of life as an adult. Design and setting: Prospective cohort study. Participants: 1) 7,222 members of the Copenhagen Perinatal Birth Cohort 1959-61 (31-33 years), 2) 9,006 mothers and their 8,820 children born in Copenhagen 1959-1961. Main outcome measures: Global QOL measured by SEQOL (self evaluation of quality of life) containing eight global QOL measures: Well-being,

---

[*] Correspondence: Søren Ventegodt, MD, MMedSci, MSc, Director, Quality of Life Research Center, Classensgade 11C, 1 sal, DK-2100 Copenhagen O, Denmark. Tel: +45-33-141113; Fax: +45-33-141123; E-mail: ventegodt@livskvalitet.org

life-satisfaction, happiness, fulfilment of needs, experience of temporal and spatial domains, expression of life's potentials, and objective factors. Results: Mother's use of psychopharmacological drugs during pregnancy had a significant, negative impact on the child's quality of life 33 years later compared to all other drugs (excepts analgesics) and no drugs. Conclusions: Maternal use of psychopharmacological drugs was negatively associated with the child's quality of life at long-term follow-up, making this group of drugs suspicious for functionally damaging the developing foetus. There might be a problem with confounders but the many statistical factors included in this study makes analysis difficult. To avoid the drugs causing harm we warn pregnant women against taking psychopharmacological drugs, and recommend the use of psychotherapy or holistic therapy (CHM) for psychological, psychiatric, and existential problems in stead.

Introduction

The Copenhagen Perinatal Birth Cohort 1959-61 has followed 8,820 children since their birth (1). During pregnancy it was noted what kind of drugs the mothers used, and after 33 years the quality of life was examined by the validated quality of life questionnaire SEQOL (self evaluation of quality of life) (2). We were able to identify 7,220 of the children after 33 years and 4,500 answered the questionnaire sufficiently.

The concept of quality of life (QOL) has become an important topic both in the health field, social welfare and the political debate. The present study was conducted to investigate the long-term effects on the quality of life on the children 33 years later of the use psychopharmacological and other drugs taken by the mother during pregnancy due to mental pain. We know from other similar studies that drugs can affect the foetus negatively (3-5), but to our knowledge the long-term effect of maternal use of psychopharmacological drugs of the child's quality of life as an adult has never been tested before.

Recently a meta-analysis documented that psychotherapy in general is more efficient that psychiatric treatment as usual (TAU) (6), which has motivated us to re-evaluate our first interpretation of the empirical results (7).

Our study

To explore the association between quality of life and the various different indicators, it was necessary to create the validated SEQOL questionnaire that could describe the global quality of life of the persons studied (2). SEQOL is a self-administered questionnaire with items rated on a five-point Likert scale. For validation SEQOL was send to 2,460 persons aged 18-88 years randomly selected from the Danish Central Person Register (CPR-Register) together with the Nottingham Health profile (NHP), Sickness Impact Factor (SIP), and the test-retest reliability correlation was > 0.8, Cronbach's alpha was 0.75, correlation (r) to NHP was 0,49, to SIP 0.27 (P<0.05). Adjustment for health status made the correlation to SIP stronger among the sick (r=0.41). For SEQOL 111 respondents were needed to detect 3% difference in QOL. SEQOL is thus valid as it shows a high level of reliability, sensitivity and consistency. For the calculation of the global QOL, 113 of the questions are used. The rest is control questions and questions giving more information about health status, sexuality, philosophy of life, life style, self-perception, and social circumstances. The principle of SEQOL is that of a hierarchy of factors, adding up to an abstract total QOL.

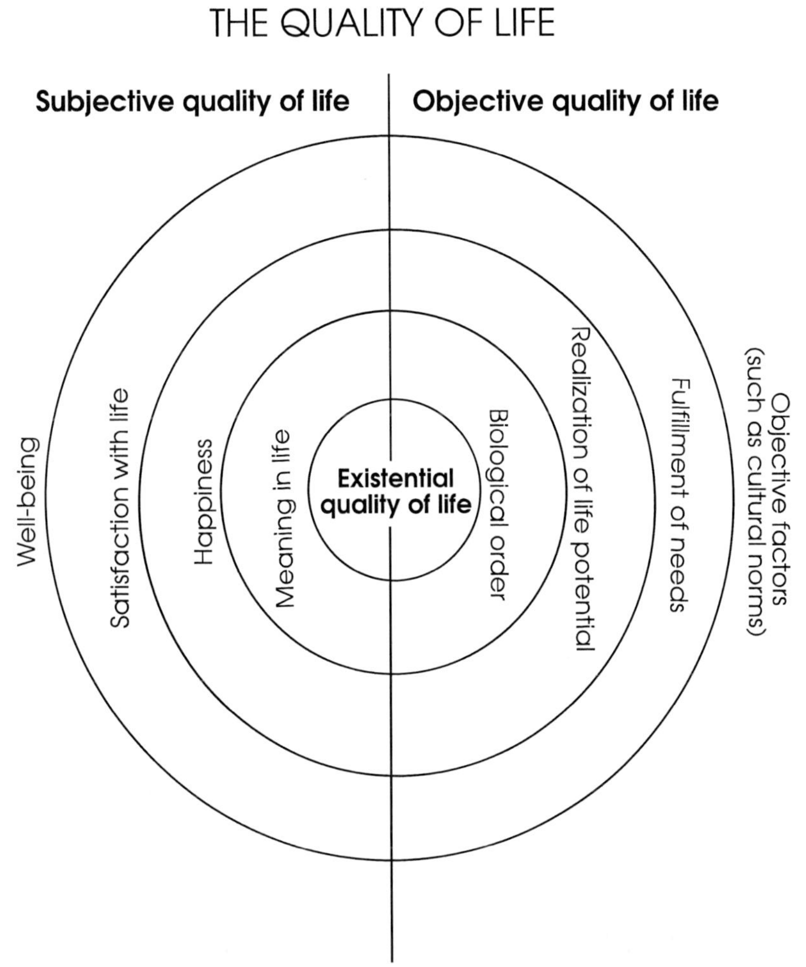

Figure 1. The integrative (IQOL) theory of the quality of life. The individual can best be compared to a green apple with red patches (a subjective and an objective quality of life, respectively at the surface of an individual's existence) with a hidden nucleus (humanity's inner depth). When this picture is combined with the picture of humanity as an onion with a number of layers between the surface and the nucleus, the taxonomy underlying the quality-of-life analysis is achieved. Between life's surface and its inexpressible depth lies well-being, satisfaction, harmony and meaning and deep concord (8).

These measures are showed below (sample questions from the questionnaire included):

Subjective measures

1. Immediate, self-experienced well-being ("How are you feeling?")
2. Life satisfaction ("How satisfying is your life?")
3. Happiness ("How happy are you at present?")

Existential measures

4. Fulfilment of needs (e.g., "How well are your social needs fulfilled?")
5. Experience of life's temporal domains (e.g., "How do you feel when you are at home?")
6. Experience of life's spatial domains ("How satisfied are you with [each of five domains: self, partner, family, friends, community]"?)
7. Expression of life's potentials [to which extent are they fulfilled]

Objective measure

8. Objective factors [income, status, work etc.]

The cohort included 7,222 persons from the Copenhagen Perinatal Birth Cohort and the results show the connection between an early life factor and the quality of life of the child 31-33 years later.

Our findings

Table 1 shows the association between mother's use of psychopharmacological drugs and the child's quality of life as adult.

Table 1 gives the data on Mother's use of psychopharmacological drugs (not barbiturates) and the child's integrated quality of life 33 years later:

- Mothers use of psychopharmacological drugs 1st month of pregnancy, five days in a row
- Mothers use of psychopharmacological drugs 1st month, five days in a row
- Mothers use of psychopharmacological drugs 2nd month, five days in a row
- Mothers use of psychopharmacological drugs 3rd month, five days in a row
- Mothers use of psychopharmacological drugs 2. Trimester, five days in a row
- Mothers use of psychopharmacological drugs 3. trimester, five days in a row
- Mothers use of psychopharmacological drugs last month, five days in a row
- Mothers use of psychopharmacological drugs at least 1 time during pregnancy

We found a significant association between quality of life and mother's use of psychopharmacological drugs during pregnancy, but we also found all other drugs – except the analgesic drugs - did not show this association. If the mother used psychopharmacological drugs only once during pregnancy, we found that the child's total I-QOL was significantly below average. Interestingly we see that the more developed the foetus is, the more damage is happening to the child.

Table 1. Psychopharmacological (not including barbiturates e.g.)

	Immediate self-experienced well-being		Life satisfaction		Happiness		Fullfilment of needs		Experience of objective temporary domains		Experience of objective spatial domains		Expression of life's potentials		Objective factors		Test (p-value)	Total IQOL
	%	n	%	n	%	n	%	n	%	n	%	n	%	n	%	n		%
First month	69,2	73	66,7	73	63,7	73	68,1	65	74,4	72	64,0	72	60,2	74	69,9	72	NS	67,7
Second month	69,6	100	67,4	100	64,4	100	68,1	88	74,7	100	64,7	98	59,4	100	70,8	97	NS	68,2
Third month	68,9	132	67,1	132	64,2	132	67,8	120	74,2	131	64,9	130	59,5	132	71,8	129	NS	68,4
2 trimester	70,6	178	68,9	178	66,3	178	68,2	160	75,1	174	66,5	169	60,6	174	72,9	172	NS	69,7
3 trimester	68,4	205	66,2	205	63,8	204	67,3	180	73,6	202	65,3	194	59,0	202	70,6	199	0.0009**	67,7
Last month	68,6	225	66,4	225	63,4	225	66,7	202	73,7	221	65,5	216	59,0	223	71,0	219	0.0020**	67,8
One time	70,1	392	68,1	392	65,1	391	67,7	351	74,6	386	66,2	378	60,1	389	72,3	379	0.0301*	69,1
None	72,0	2105	69,4	2106	66,1	2106	68,4	1929	74,9	2080	67,2	2048	61,8	2096	72,8	2060	NS	70,0

This most strongly suggest a biological mechanism; if the use of psychopharmacological drugs were an indication of mother's poor mental health, personality problem, or chronically mental illness, we would have seen a significant associations between the use of psychopharmacological drugs and child's QOL also when the drugs were used early in pregnancy. We do not find it likely that the use of drugs signifies a birth depression, as this normally first manifest itself after the birth of the child.

No other drugs – except for analgesic drugs - on the long list recorded by the researchers in 1959-61 were associated with a similar lowering of the quality of life: Antihistamines, anti-epileptics, barbiturates, antibiotics, chemotherapy, hormones, anti-hormones, diuretics, and "other drugs".

Discussion

The data presented in this paper suggest that the foetus is biologically vulnerable to maternal use of psychopharmacological drugs, especially during third trimester, where the brain develops mostly. More modest damage might also happen to the foetus in the first two trimesters as we find that only one single episode of using psychopharmacological drugs was significantly connected with compromised quality of life of the child 33 years later. There is a problem with confounders in this study, as we have included so many factors that the confounder analysis for this reason alone gives insignificant results (a problem similar to mass-significance, just opposite). We therefore cannot completely rule out that what we see is a true biological effect of psychopharmachological drugs, and we therefore find that we for ethical reasons (Hippocrates: First do not harm) most warn pregnant women against using drugs, as psychotherapy is as efficient, and seemingly less harmful.

Even if we accept the result as significant, there are still several alternative interpretations of the data: 1) Maternal mental disease is in itself affecting the unborn child, 2) Mother using these drugs is more likely to be mentally ill during the child's upbringing and 3) The use of psychopharmacological drugs is an indicator for poverty or other negative life circumstances affecting the child negatively. These hypotheses are very appealing, but seem to be in conflict with the fact that there is a very large dependency of the trimester in which the psychopharmacological drugs were taken – a pattern not seen with the drugs i.e. analgesics. Presumably a mother being insane in first or second trimester is as likely to be mentally ill during the child's upbringing as is a mother being insane in the third. Such arguments have lead to our reinterpretation of the empirical data.

Conclusions

For the first time it has been possible prospectively to study in details the effect of the pregnant mother's use of psychopharmacological drugs on the quality of life 33 years later; unfortunately we have collected too many factors to be able to conveniently use standard statistics. If the drugs cause many small damages to the developing foetus these will not be visible in themselves, but when we measure them all together in an integrated QOL measure looking both at subjective, objective and existential factors, they might become visible.

The data suggest a significant, negative influence on the child's permanent quality of life, if the mother used psychopharmacological drugs during pregnancy for mental pain. The damage seemed to be largest late in pregnancy, which not surprisingly indicates damage to the foetal developing brain. We recommend that pregnant women only use psychopharmacological drugs when psychotherapy or holistic therapy (CHM) has failed to help them; fortunately recent meta-analysis has documented psychotherapy to be more efficient that standard psychiatric treatment (8).

If the developing foetus is vulnerable to psychopharmacological drugs, a fertile woman with an active sexual life should avoid using such drugs, as she never can be completely sure not to get pregnant. We recommend that pregnant women take psychopharmacological drugs only when psychotherapy or scientific, holistic therapy has failed to help.

Acknowledgments

This paper reports results from the Danish Quality of Life Population Survey, the planning and execution of which would not have been possible without the aid of Dorte Loldrup Poulsen, Jørgen Hilden and the late Bengt Zachau-Christiansen scientific work(1,9). Funds were received from several Danish Foundations, including The 1991 Pharmacy, the Goodwill, the JL, E. Danielsens and Wife's, Emmerick Meyer's, the Frimodt-Heineken, the Family Hede Nielsen's, Petrus Andersen's, C.P. Frederiksen's and the Wedell-Wedellsborgs Foundations, and IMK Almene Fond. The research was approved by the Copenhagen Ethical Committee under numbers (KF) V 100.1762/90 and (KF) 01-502/93.

References

[1] Zachau-Christiansen B. The influence of prenatal and perinatal factors on development during the first year of life with special reference to the development of signs of cerebral dysfunction. A prospective study of 9,006 pregnancies. Elsinore, DK: Poul A Andersen, 1972.

[2] Ventegodt S, Henneberg EW, Merrick J, Lindholt JS. Validation of two global and generic quality of life questionnaires for population screening: SCREENQOL and SEQOL. ScientificWorldJournal 2003;3:412–21.

[3] Shehata HA, Nelson-Piercy C. Drugs in pregnancy. Drugs to avoid. Best Pract Res Clin Obstet Gynaecol 2001;15(6):971-86.

[4] Ornoy A. The effects of alcohol and illicit drugs on the human embryo and fetus. Isr J Psychiatry Relat Sci 2002;39(2):120-32.

[5] Reinisch JM, Sanders SA, Mortensen AL, Rubin DB. In utero exposure to phenobarbital and intelligence deficits in adult men. JAMA 1995;274: 1518-25.

[6] Leichsenring F, Leibing E. Psychodynamic psychotherapy: a systematic review of techniques, indications and empirical evidence. Psychol Psychother 2007;80(Pt 2):217-28.

[7] Ventegodt S, Merrick J. Long-term effects of maternal medication on global quality of life measured with SEQOL. Results from the Copenhagen Perinatal Birth Cohort 1959-61. ScientificWorldJournal 2003;3:707-13.

[8] Ventegodt S. Measuring the quality of life. From theory to practice. Copenhagen: Forskningscentrets Forlag, 1996.

[9] Zachau-Christiansen B, Ross EM. Babies: Human development during the first Year. London: John Wiley, 1975.

IX. Acknowledgments

In: Children and Pain
Editors: P. Schofield and J. Merrick
ISBN 978-1-60876-020-6

Chapter 14

About the editors

Patricia Schofield, RGN, PhD, PGDipEd, DipN is senior lecturer at the Centre for Advanced Studies in Nursing, Department of General Practice and Primary Care, University of Aberdeen in the United Kingdom has worked in pain management since 1988. Originally as a clinical nurse specialist in Chesterfield and then as a lecturer and senior lecturer. PhD thesis on nursing interventions for the management of chronic pain and set up the first pain management course for nurses in the UK. Completed a number of post doctoral projects around pain management in older people including talking to them about their pain experiences, a systematic review and two annotated bibliographies. Served on council for the British Pain Society and recently set up a special interest group around pain in older adults. Currently working with the British Geriatric Society setting up guidelines for pain assessment in older adults and leading a group of researchers developing a number of projects around pain assessment in care homes and pain management for older adults. Several books and publications in this area of research. Co-editor of the Journal of Pain Management published by Nova Science in New York. E-mail: p.a.schofield@abdn.ac.uk

Joav Merrick, MD, MMedSci, DMSc is professor of pediatrics, child health and human development affiliated with Kentucky Children's Hospital, University of Kentucky, Lexington, United States and the Zusman Child Development Center, Division of Pediatrics, Soroka University Medical Center, Ben Gurion University, Beer-Sheva, Israel, the medical director of the Division for Mental Retardation, Ministry of Social Affairs, Jerusalem, the founder and director of the National Institute of Child Health and Human Development. Numerous publications in the field of pediatrics, child health and human development, rehabilitation, intellectual disability, disability, health, welfare, abuse, advocacy, quality of life and prevention. Received the Peter Sabroe Child Award for outstanding work on behalf of Danish Children in 1985 and the International LEGO-Prize ("The Children's Nobel Prize") for an extraordinary contribution towards improvement in child welfare and well-being in 1987. E-mail: jmerrick@zahav.net.il; Website: www.nichd-israel.com; Home-page: http://jmerrick50.googlepages.com/home

In: Children and Pain
Editors: P. Schofield and J. Merrick
ISBN 978-1-60876-020-6

Chapter 15

About the National Institute of Child Health and Human Devlopment in Israel

The National Institute of Child Health and Human Development (NICHD) in Israel was established in 1998 as a virtual institute under the auspicies of the Medical Director, Ministry of Social Affairs and Social Services in order to function as the research arm for the Office of the Medical Director. In 1998 the National Council for Child Health and Pediatrics, Ministry of Health and in 1999 the Director General and Deputy Director General of the Ministry of Health endorsed the establishment of the NICHD.

Mission

The mission of a National Institute for Child Health and Human Development in Israel is to provide an academic focal point for the scholarly interdisciplinary study of child life, health, public health, welfare, disability, rehabilitation, intellectual disability and related aspects of human development. This mission includes research, teaching, clinical work, information and public service activities in the field of child health and human development.

Service and academic activities

Over the years many activities became focused in the south of Israel due to collaboration with various professionals at the Faculty of Health Sciences (FOHS) at the Ben Gurion University of the Negev (BGU). Since 2000 an affiliation with the Zusman Child Development Center at the Pediatric Division of Soroka University Medical Center has resulted in collaboration around the establishment of the Down Syndrome Clinic at that center. In 2002 a full course on "Disability" was established at the Recanati School for Allied Professions in the Community, FOHS, BGU and twice a year seminars for specialists in family medicine. In 2005 collaboration was started with the Primary Care Unit of the faculty and disability became part of the master of public health course on "Children and society". In the academic year 2005-2006 a one semester course on "Aging with disability" was started as part of the master of science program in gerontology in our collaboration with the Center for Multidisciplinary Research in Aging.

Research activities

The affiliated staff has over the years published work from projects and research activities in this national and international collaboration. In the year 2000 the International Journal of Adolescent Medicine and Health and in 2005 the International Journal on Disability and Human development of Freund Publishing House (London and Tel Aviv), in the year 2003 the TSW-Child Health and Human Development and in 2006 the TSW-Holistic Health and Medicine of the Scientific World Journal (New York and Kirkkonummi, Finland), all peer-reviewed international journals were affiliated with the National Institute of Child Health and Human Development. From 2008 also the International Journal of Child Health and Human Development (Nova Science, New York), the International Journal of Child and Adolescent Health (Nova Science) and the Journal of Pain Management (Nova Science) affiliated.

National collaborations

Nationally the NICHD works in collaboration with the Faculty of Health Sciences, Ben Gurion University of the Negev; Department of Physical Therapy, Sackler School of Medicine, Tel Aviv University; Autism Center, Assaf HaRofeh Medical Center; National Rett and PKU Centers at Chaim Sheba Medical Center, Tel HaShomer; Department of Physiotherapy, Haifa University; Department of Education, Bar Ilan University, Ramat Gan, Faculty of Social Sciences and Health Sciences; College of Judea and Samaria in Ariel and recently also collaborations has been established with the Division of Pediatrics at Hadassah, Center for Pediatric Chronic Illness, Har HaZofim in Jerusalem.

International collaborations

Internationally with the Department of Disability and Human Development, College of Applied Health Sciences, University of Illinois at Chicago; Strong Center for Developmental Disabilities, Golisano Children's Hospital at Strong, University of Rochester School of Medicine and Dentistry, New York; Centre on Intellectual Disabilities, University of Albany, New York; Centre for Chronic Disease Prevention and Control, Health Canada, Ottawa; Chandler Medical Center and Children's Hospital, Kentucky Children's Hospital, Section of Adolescent Medicine, University of Kentucky, Lexington; Chronic Disease Prevention and Control Research Center, Baylor College of Medicine, Houston, Texas; Division of Neuroscience, Department of Psychiatry, Columbia University, New York; Institute for the Study of Disadvantage and Disability, Atlanta; Center for Autism and Related Disorders,

Department Psychiatry, Children's Hospital Boston, Boston; Department of Paediatrics, Child Health and Adolescent Medicine, Children's Hospital at Westmead, Westmead, Australia; International Centre for the Study of Occupational and Mental Health, Düsseldorf, Germany; Centre for Advanced Studies in Nursing, Department of General Practice and Primary Care, University of Aberdeen, Aberdeen, United Kingdom; Quality of Life Research Center, Copenhagen, Denmark; Nordic School of Public Health, Gottenburg, Sweden, Scandinavian Institute of Quality of Working Life, Oslo, Norway; Centre for Quality of Life of the Hong Kong Institute of Asia-Pacific Studies and School of Social Work, Chinese University, Hong Kong.

Targets

Our focus is on research, international collaborations, clinical work, teaching and policy in health, disability and human development and to establish the NICHD as a permanent institute at one of the residential care centers for persons with intellectual disability in Israel in order to conduct model research and together with the four university schools of public health/medicine in Israel establish a national master and doctoral program in disability and human development at the institute to secure the next generation of professionals working in this often non-prestigious/low-status field of work. For this project we need your support. We are looking for all kinds of support and eventually an endowment.

Contact

Professor Joav Merrick, MD, MMedSci, DMSc
Medical Director, Division for Mental Retardation
Ministry of Social Affairs, POBox 1260
IL-91012 Jerusalem, Israel
E-mail: jmerrick@internet-zahav.net
Website: www.nichd-israel.com;

Index

B

C

D

E

F

I

J

K

L

M

P

Q

R

S

T

U

V

W

Y